Clinical Practical Procedures for Junior Doctors

Commissioning Editor: Timothy Horne
Development Editor: Ailsa Laing
Project Manager: Anne Dickie/Sukanthi Sukumar
Designer: Kirsteen Wright
Illustration Manager: Merlyn Harvey
Illustrator: Ethan Danielson

CHURCHILL'S POCKETBOOKS OF

Clinical Practical Procedures for Junior Doctors

Nisha Patel BSc(Hons) MBBS MRCP
Specialist Registrar in Gastroenterology,
Chelsea and Westminster Hospital NHS Trust, London, UK

Daniel Knight BSc(Hons) MBBS MRCP
Specialist Registrar in Cardiology,
Royal Free Hampstead NHS Trust, London, UK

Edited by

Mark Palazzo MB FRCA FRCP MD
Chief of Service, Directorate of Critical Care Medicine
and Anaesthetics, Imperial College Healthcare NHS Trust,
Charing Cross Hospital, London, UK

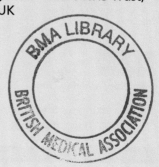

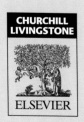

CHURCHILL
LIVINGSTONE

ELSEVIER

EDINBURGH   LONDON   NEW YORK   OXFORD
PHILADELPHIA   ST LOUIS   SYDNEY   TORONTO   2009

CHURCHILL
LIVINGSTONE
ELSEVIER

First published 2009, © Elsevier Limited. All rights reserved.

ISBN 978-0-443-06806-5

British Library Cataloguing in Publication Data
A catalogue record for this book is available from the British Library

Library of Congress Cataloging in Publication Data
A catalog record for this book is available from the Library of Congress

Notice
Knowledge and best practice in this field are constantly changing. As new research and experience broaden our knowledge, changes in practice, treatment and drug therapy may become necessary or appropriate. Readers are advised to check the most current information provided (i) on procedures featured or (ii) by the manufacturer of each product to be administered, to verify the recommended dose or formula, the method and duration of administration, and contraindications. It is the responsibility of the practitioner, relying on their own experience and knowledge of the patient, to make diagnoses, to determine dosages and the best treatment for each individual patient, and to take all appropriate safety precautions. To the fullest extent of the law, neither the Publisher nor the Authors assume any liability for any injury and/or damage to persons or property arising out of or related to any use of the material contained in this book.

The Publisher

ELSEVIER your source for books, journals and multimedia in the health sciences

www.elsevierhealth.com

Working together to grow libraries in developing countries

www.elsevier.com | www.bookaid.org | www.sabre.org

ELSEVIER   BOOK AID International   Sabre Foundation

The Publisher's policy is to use paper manufactured from sustainable forests

Printed in China

CONTENTS

After the celebrations of graduating from medical school, the reality of starting out as an inexperienced junior doctor can be particularly stressful. As first year doctors ourselves not so long ago, being left on the wards to do that 'urgent lumbar puncture' or 'quick ascitic tap' was a dauntingly familiar story. Clinical practical procedures are widely taught on models in medical schools. However, putting this theoretical training into clinical practice in your junior years can be particularly disconcerting. While providing a basic foundation upon which to learn procedures, models can never translate to the reality of performing them on a patient under difficult circumstances, for example, on an acutely unwell patient in the middle of the night. Of the multiple factors involved in this stressful time, we hope this book alleviates those associated with performing clinical practical procedures.

We aim to provide you with a valuable tool and reference point when asked to perform these clinical procedures. As one of the *Churchill's Pocketbooks* series it can be conveniently carried in your bag or pocket. Related practical procedures are grouped under the relevant system in a recognizable 'ABC' approach, making it easier to find a procedure quickly. Each chapter starts with the origins of the procedure, its indications and potential complications to be aware of before you start. After all, you must know what to explain to the patient pre-procedure and what to prepare for should things go wrong. The procedures are outlined in an easy-to-read manner using a step-by-step approach, with abundant diagrams and clinical photographs to complement the text. Chapters finish with post-procedure care, how to process investigations and the basics of their interpretation. Performing the procedures successfully is not the end-point of course; you must know what to do with the cerebrospinal fluid or ascitic fluid you managed to obtain. Tip Boxes are present throughout the chapters to highlight useful points regarding the procedure, common pitfalls and improvements to your delivery.

We hope you enjoy this book and use it to improve your clinical procedural skills, giving you confidence to perform them on the wards and on-call.

ACKNOWLEDGEMENTS

We would like to express our gratitude to the patients who kindly agreed to have their clinical procedures photographed. Without their willingness to assist, this educational resource would not be possible. We thank Dr Patrick Doyle for his help and expertise. Thank you to Chris Priest, Nicola Webster and Philippa Hutton at Medical Illustration UK Ltd for their help with the medical photography. We thank Christopher Knight for his assistance. We would also like to thank all the staff at Elsevier for their help with this project.

Finally, we would like to thank our parents and partners, Kinesh and Amy, for their patience, understanding and support in completing this book.

AIRWAY CARE WITH SIMPLE DEVICES

The first procedure used for airway control was probably tracheostomy. Pedro Virgili (1699–1776) from Cadiz used it for the relief of quinsy, but its popularity was assured by its success in the management of diphtheria. The first to use it in the UK for diphtheria was George Martine (1702–1741). The eminent surgeon Sir William MacEwen (1848–1924) first performed intubation of the upper laryngeal orifice and trachea in 1878 as an alternative to tracheostomy, again for the management of life-threatening airway obstruction due to diphtheria.

INTRODUCTION

The assessment of airway patency and its safeguard are essential skills for acute life-support. Recognition of an obstructed airway is initially manifested by a combination of ventilatory efforts and airway sounds reflecting airflow turbulence, which become relatively quickly complicated by the signs of inadequate respiratory function such as cyanosis, tachycardia, and loss of consciousness.

VENTILATORY EFFORT

- Increased accessory muscle activity.
- Mouth opening with each inspiratory effort.
- Suprasternal and chest wall indrawing rather than chest expansion with every inspiratory effort.

AIRWAY SOUNDS

- Stridor – a harsh noise produced on aggressively trying to inspire air to overcome an obstruction at or above the level of the larynx.
- Wheeze – a sound heard at the mouth or on chest auscultation during expiration.
  — The pitch of the wheeze may be described as polyphonic, commonly observed in asthma and chronic obstructive airways disease. This sound suggests many

airways of differing calibre are simultaneously in varying states of compromise due to spasm and/or narrowing secondary to mucosal inflammation. The wheeze of asthma is easily heard at the mouth and confirmed by chest auscultation.
— Wheeze with a single sound (monophonic) particularly located in just one area indicates obstruction of a single bronchus, e.g. by tumour. The fixed wheeze (also called rhonchus) of bronchial obstruction is not e asily heard at the mouth.
- Crowing – a loud sound heard with every inspiration not dissimilar to stridor and suggests turbulent flow due to flow through a narrow orifice commonly heard during laryngeal spasm.
- Gurgling – the sound of air bubbling through liquid or semi-solid debris in the upper airways is mostly heard during inspiration.
- Snoring – a long inspiratory sound associated with partial occlusion of the pharynx by the tongue or soft palate.

Tip Box
An obstructed airway is a clinical emergency. If you are not confident in managing the airway, call for *immediate anaesthetic assistance*.

AIRWAY MANAGEMENT

AIRWAY CLEARANCE

Look inside the oral cavity and remove any vomitus, debris or foreign bodies with the following devices:

- Yankauer sucker (Fig. 1.1A) – a rigid suction device that is attached to a vacuum collection system for facilitating removal of liquid or semi-solid debris from the oropharynx.
- Magill's forceps (Fig. 1.1B) – in the acute setting these are used to remove foreign bodies from the oral cavity. Magill's forceps are also used to guide nasogastric tubes into the oesophagus under direct vision and to place pharyngeal packs.

BASIC AIRWAY TECHNIQUES

- Head tilt, chin lift (Fig. 1.2): avoid if suspected cervical spine trauma – place one hand on the patient's forehead and the fingertips of your other hand under the patient's chin. Whilst gently tilting the head back lift the patient's chin to open the airway.

- Jaw thrust (Fig. 1.3) – this is the technique of choice in the presence of suspected cervical spine injury. Place the index fingers behind the angle of the mandible and apply steady upwards pressure to bring the mandible forwards. Slightly open the mouth by downwards displacement of the chin with your thumbs.

Tip Box

Suspected C-spine injury – The jaw thrust is the technique of choice in such patients for basic airway management, with manual in-line stabilization of the head and neck performed by a second operator. However, the primary and over-riding objective in all cases is the maintenance of a patent airway as an obstructed airway is the most immediate threat to life.

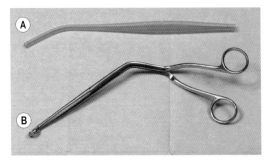

Fig. 1.1 (A) Yankauer sucker. The curved nature of the device allows its insertion into the upper pharynx. (B) Magill's forceps. The angle in the forceps enables them to be used with the handles out of the line of vision of the operator.

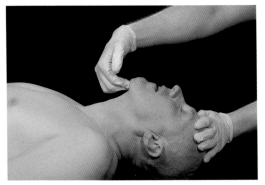

Fig. 1.2 Head tilt, chin lift.

SECTION 1 **Airway and breathing**

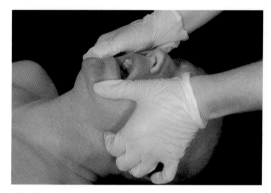

Fig. 1.3   Jaw thrust manoeuvre.

AIRWAY ADJUNCTS

Oropharyngeal (Guedel) airways

Curved plastic tubes with a flange that fit between the tongue and hard palate thereby maintaining a patent oropharynx (Fig. 1.4). If glossopharyngeal or laryngeal reflexes are present, the insertion of a Guedel airway may stimulate vomiting or laryngospasm, respectively. Hence, these should only be inserted in the comatose patient.

The size of the oropharyngeal airway is that size which matches:

- the distance between the incisors to the angle of the jaw (Fig. 1.5A) or
- the distance between the corner of the mouth to the tragus (Fig. 1.5B).

See Fig. 1.6 for how to introduce the Guedel airway. Using this technique minimizes the risk of pushing the tongue backwards.

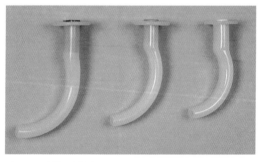

Fig. 1.4   Oropharyngeal (Guedel) airways.

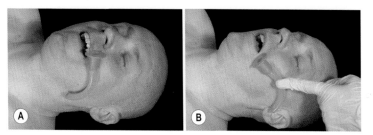

Fig. 1.5 Judging what size of Guedel airway to choose. (A) Distance between the incisors to the angle of the jaw. (B) Distance from the angle of the mouth to the tragus.

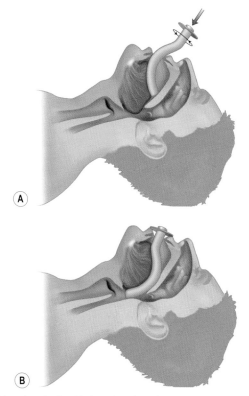

Fig. 1.6 (A) Introduce the Guedel airway into the oral cavity in the upside-down position. (B) As the airway passes below the hard palate rotate it through 180 degrees while advancing into the oropharynx.

- A suction catheter can be passed down the oropharyngeal airway to clear liquid or semi-solid debris.
- Once the Guedel airway is placed make sure the flange is not sitting proud outside the mouth. The airway can be kept in place with your thumbs and this manoeuvre may need to be combined with jaw thrust to ensure complete patency.
- The chest should be moving freely with no evidence of upper airway obstruction, such as suprasternal recession with ventilatory effort. If in doubt recheck the placement of the Guedel airway.

Nasopharyngeal airways

These provide a patent nasopharyngeal airway in patients in whom an oropharyngeal airway is unsuitable, either because the patient is not deeply unconscious or because of lack of oral access (e.g. trismus or maxillofacial trauma) (Fig. 1.7).

- The size of the nasopharyngeal airway is given in millimetres according to the internal tube diameter. The size of the airway required is the one in which the internal diameter corresponds to the diameter of the patient's little finger, commonly approximately 6 mm for females and 7 mm for males.
- Having lubricated the airway with a water-based jelly, it is inserted into the nostril bevel-first and passed in a posterior direction with a slight twisting motion.
- The airway should be inserted such that the flange should lie at the level of the nostril. A safety pin is placed through the flange prior to insertion in order to prevent the airway slipping beyond the nares.

Note that patients on anticoagulants or platelet-function-modifying drugs may bleed during this procedure. This is a necessary risk if the airway is compromised. A suction catheter can be passed down the nasopharyngeal airway to clear liquid or semi-solid debris, although care should be taken as this can cause the patient to gag and subsequently vomit.

Tip Box

Nasopharyngeal airways are contraindicated in suspected base of skull fracture, the signs of which include:

- CSF rhinorrhoea or otorrhoea
- 'Racoon eyes' – bruising of the orbits resulting from blood collecting from the fracture site
- 'Battle's sign' – bruising behind the ears from blood collecting from the fracture site

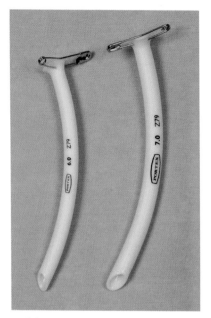

Fig. 1.7   Nasopharyngeal airways.

Laryngeal mask airway (LMA)

Whilst an LMA (Fig. 1.8) is not as definitive as an endotracheal tube, it is a reliable airway adjunct that can be used by medical professionals with a range of experience levels.

- Prior to using the LMA check the integrity of the cuff by inflating it with the required volume of air stipulated on the device.
- Fully deflate the cuff and liberally apply lubricating jelly to the **outer face** of the cuff.
- Hold the LMA like a pen and insert into the oral cavity tip-first and with the aperture pointing downwards (Fig. 1.9A).
- Advance the LMA with the upper surface against the palate. Upon reaching the pharyngeal wall press the LMA backwards and downwards around the corner of the pharynx. The operator will feel resistance once the LMA is located in the back of the hypopharynx (Fig. 1.9B).

SECTION 1 Airway and breathing

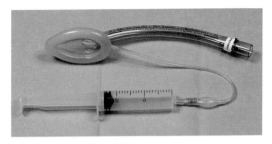

Fig. 1.8 Laryngeal mask airway with cuff inflated.

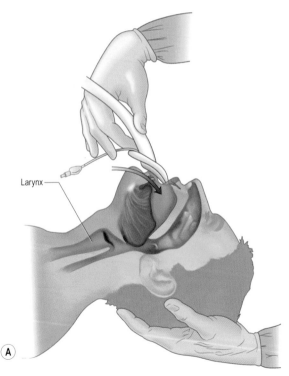

Larynx

(A)

Fig. 1.9 (A) Hold the LMA like a pen and insert with the aperture pointing downwards.

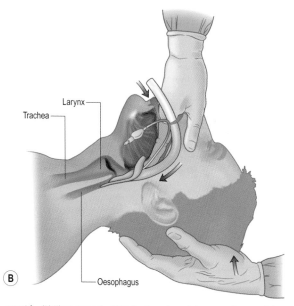

Larynx

Trachea

Oesophagus

(B)

Fig. 1.9—cont'd (B) Then press the LMA backwards and downwards around the corner of the pharynx. Resistance will be felt once the LMA is located in the back of the hypopharynx.

- Inflate the cuff with the volume of air stated on the device from a syringe.
- Auscultate the chest bilaterally for air entry and inspect the chest wall for bilateral movement. If air entry is not noted bilaterally then the LMA should be deflated and immediately removed. Ventilation should subsequently recommence with a bag–valve–mask until it is suitable to either retry with an LMA or an anaesthetist attends to place an endotracheal tube.

Tip Box

Take care to avoid lacerating the patient's upper lip against their teeth whilst inserting the LMA.

Endotracheal tube (ETT)

Only to be considered by personnel with required training (hence not covered in this text).

OXYGEN DELIVERY

Venturi mask valves

These devices allow controlled oxygen therapy for self-ventilating patients with chronic obstructive airways disease (Fig. 1.10 and Table 1.1). They attach to a face mask and oxygen tubing and deliver oxygen at a predetermined rate indicated on the valve. Depending upon the aperture size on the valve device, a fixed fractional inspired oxygen concentration (FiO_2) is subsequently delivered to the mask. It should be remembered, however, that in the acute setting of respiratory distress, first priority must be given to the management of hypoxia using high FiO_2 delivery systems such as the non-rebreathe mask.

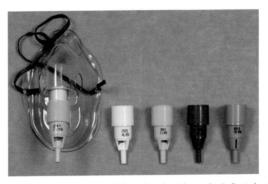

Fig. 1.10 Venturi mask valves. Oxygen delivered to the valve at the indicated rate will subsequently deliver the stipulated FiO_2 to the patient.

TABLE 1.1 Venturi mask key		
Venturi valve colour	*Flow rate (L/min)*	*FiO_2 (%)*
Blue	2	24
White	4	28
Yellow	8	35
Red	10	40
Green	15	60

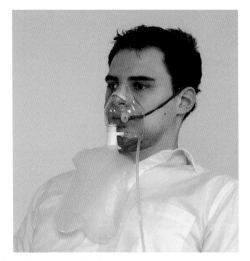

Fig. 1.11   Patient using a 'non-rebreathe' mask.

Non-rebreathe oxygen mask

Oxygen is delivered via tubing at 10–15 L/min to the reservoir bag, which is initially filled by manually occluding the one-way valve. Having attached the mask to the face (see Fig. 1.11), oxygen is inspired by the patient from the reservoir bag thereby increasing the FiO_2. Expired air escapes to the atmosphere via the mask apertures, and in doing so closes the one-way valve between the mask and the reservoir bag. This allows the reservoir bag to automatically refill with oxygen between breaths, and separates inhaled and exhaled gases (hence a 'non-rebreathe' mask).

Bag–valve–mask device (Fig. 1.12)

This three-part device is indicated for use in patients who are either apnoeic or who are not ventilating adequately. The three parts include:

- a reservoir bag that can be filled with oxygen
- a ventilating bag that, when compressed, passes oxygen towards the patient
- a one-way valve between the ventilating bag and the face mask, which permits the flow of inspiratory gas to the patient but closes to expired gas from the patient, thus allowing only the contents of the reservoir bag to serve as inhaled gas.

The bag–valve apparatus can not only be connected to a face mask, but also to a laryngeal mask or endotracheal tube to deliver ventilatory support. If the bag–valve is connected to a face mask it is easier to have two operators (Fig. 1.13). One operator

SECTION 1 **Airway and breathing**

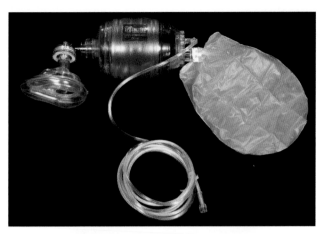

Fig. 1.12 Bag–valve–mask device.

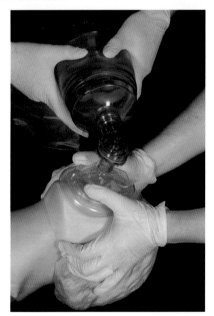

Fig. 1.13 Using the bag–valve–mask device requires two operators. One operator ensures satisfactory and secure placement of the tight-fitting mask with both hands whilst tilting the patient's head and lifting their chin; the other squeezes the contents of the bag, again using two hands.

ensures satisfactory and secure placement of the tight fitting–mask whilst tilting the patient's head and lifting their chin, the other squeezes the contents of the bag with two hands (see Fig. 1.13).

100% oxygen can be delivered by the apparatus by attaching a fast-flow oxygen supply (10 L/min) to the reservoir bag. Gases breathed out are vented through the one-way valve to the atmosphere.

CHAPTER 2

PEAK EXPIRATORY FLOW RATE MEASUREMENT AND SPIROMETRY

The spirometer was invented by physician John Hutchison (1811–1861) in 1846. The peak flow meter was introduced into clinical use around 1960.

INTRODUCTION

Peak expiratory flow rate (PEFR) and bedside spirometry are simple and cheap non-invasive measures of ventilatory function. A peak flow meter (Fig. 2.1) measures the fastest rate of expiratory airflow in litres per minute. Peak flow meters come in various guises, but they all serve the same function.

Spirometry (Fig. 2.2) also measures expiratory airflow, but provides extra information including the forced expiratory volume in one second (FEV_1), the forced vital capacity (FVC) and the FEV_1/FVC ratio. The value of this ratio can be indicative of obstructive or restrictive ventilatory deficits.

INDICATIONS

- Any condition that requires monitoring of ventilatory function, either acute, e.g. acute exacerbation of asthma, Guillain-Barré syndrome, or chronic, e.g. asthma.
- Pre-operative assessment of ventilatory function and capacity.

SECTION 1 Airway and breathing

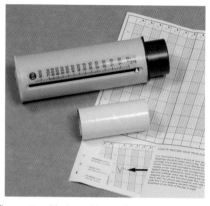

Fig. 2.1 A peak flow meter with disposable mouthpiece.

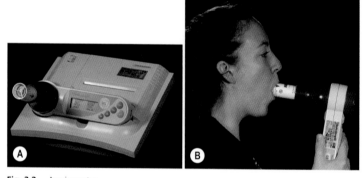

Fig. 2.2 A spirometer.

CONTRAINDICATIONS

Spirometry is a safe and non-invasive test. However, performing PEFR measurement or spirometry does increase intra-thoracic, intra-abdominal and intra-ocular pressures. Therefore, spirometry does carry a small risk to individuals with certain co-morbidities, and so these can be regarded as **relative** contraindications:

- lack of consent
- unstable angina, recent myocardial infarction or stroke

- recent pneumothorax
- recent ocular surgery
- recent abdominal surgery
- undiagnosed haemoptysis.

EQUIPMENT

- Peak flow meter and clean mouthpiece.
- Peak flow chart.
- Bedside spirometer (with attached graph paper if a manual tracing).
- Bronchodilator inhaler (with spacer if required) for reversibility testing.

PRACTICAL PROCEDURE – PEFR

Tip Box
Patients who are taking inhaled bronchodilators may give unreliable measurements if testing is not synchronized with their dosing regimen. If the patient is taking inhaled bronchodilators, the scheduled regular dose prior to performing PEFR measurement or spirometry should be omitted in order to give valid pre- and post-bronchodilator measurements.

Tip Box
Demonstrate to the patient how to perform the procedure prior to their attempt.

- Obtain consent.
- Check that the pointer is at zero and that a clean mouthpiece is in place.
- The patient should preferably stand upright, holding the peak flow meter with the fingers away from the pointer.
- Ask the patient to inhale a large breath through their mouth, then place their lips around the mouthpiece forming a tight seal, and then breathe out as hard and fast as possible.

Tip Box

Compare this to an example such as blowing out candles on a cake, and emphasize that it is the speed of the blow that is being measured.

- Ensuring correct technique, repeat the measurement three times in total and document the best measurement.
- If appropriate, repeat the above process approximately 10 min after inhaling a bronchodilator.
- Dispose of the mouthpiece.
- Document PEFR on a peak flow chart (Fig. 2.3) pre- and post-bronchodilator at both morning and night (looking for diurnal variation, a hallmark of asthma being so-called 'morning dips').
- Compare the patient's PEFR with the ideal PEFR for their height (Fig. 2.4).

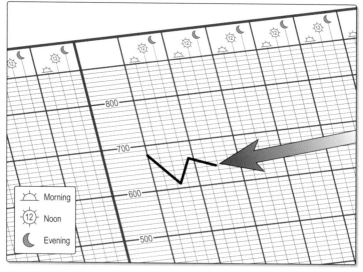

Fig. 2.3 PEFR chart, for recording results at standard intervals throughout the day.

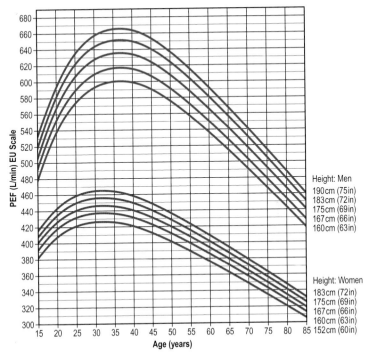

Fig. 2.4   Normal peak flow values adjusted for height (adapted by C. Clarke from Nunn AJ, Gregg I. BMJ 1989;298:1068–70).

PRACTICAL PROCEDURE – SPIROMETRY

- Obtain consent.
- Check that a clean mouthpiece is in place.
- The patient should preferably stand upright. A noseclip should be used to prevent nasal air flow.
- Ask the patient to inhale a large breath through their mouth, then place their lips around the mouthpiece forming a tight seal, and then breathe out as hard and fast and as long as possible until their lungs are completely empty.

Tip Box

Compare this to an example such as blowing out candles on a cake but encourage the patient to keep blowing for as long as possible.

SECTION 1 **Airway and breathing**

- Ensuring correct technique, repeat the measurement three times in total.
- If appropriate, repeat the above process approximately 10 min after inhaling a bronchodilator.
- Dispose of the mouthpiece.
- Document the procedure clearly in the medical notes.

INTERPRETING THE SPIROMETRY RESULTS

Spirometry using a traditional vitalograph provides a volume–time curve (Fig. 2.5).

- FEV_1 (forced expiratory volume in one second) = the maximal volume of air exhaled within one second.
- FVC (forced vital capacity) = the total volume of air exhaled in one breath.
- Ratio of FEV_1/FVC = the proportion of the total air in the lungs that can be exhaled in one second (normally 70–80%).

These values vary characteristically in different disease states of the lung (Table 2.1).
More modern, sophisticated spirometry equipment displays the data as a flow–volume loop (Fig. 2.6). The shape of the flow–volume loop will also vary characteristically in different disease states of the lung (Fig. 2.7).
In some cases, a mixed obstructive/restrictive picture will be evident, either due to co-existent obstructive and restrictive conditions (e.g. asthma and interstitial lung disease, Table 2.2) or due to conditions displaying both obstructive and restrictive characteristics (e.g. cystic fibrosis).

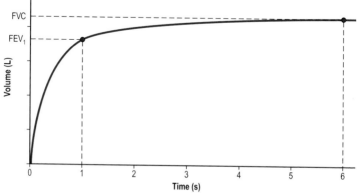

Fig. 2.5 Volume–time curve from a vitalograph.

TABLE 2.1 Spirometry results in obstructive versus restrictive states

	Normal (70 kg man)	Obstructive defect	Restrictive defect
FEV$_1$ (L)	4	⇊	↓
FVC (L)	5	↓	⇊
FEV$_1$/FVC	70–80%	↓ (<70%)	Normal or ↑ (>80%)

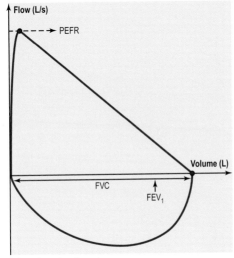

Fig. 2.6   Flow–volume loop in spirometry.

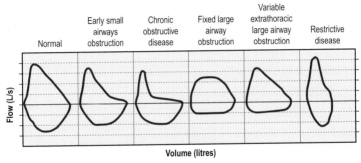

Fig. 2.7   Shapes of flow–volume loops in different respiratory diseases.

TABLE 2.2 Examples of obstructive and restrictive lung defects

Obstructive	Restrictive
Asthma	Thoracic wall deformities
Chronic obstructive airways disease –emphysema –chronic bronchitis	Interstitial lung disease –pulmonary fibrosis –sarcoidosis
Bronchiectasis	Pulmonary oedema
	Neuromuscular disease (e.g. Guillain-Barré syndrome)
	Recurrent pulmonary emboli
	Lymphangitis carcinomatosa

CHAPTER 3

PLEURAL ASPIRATION (OF FLUID OR AIR)

INTRODUCTION

Pleural aspiration of fluid or air is a bedside technique that can be performed for diagnostic and/or therapeutic purposes.

INDICATIONS

- Diagnostic aspiration of pleural fluid.
- Therapeutic aspiration of pleural effusion (better done by placing a drain; see Chapter 4).
- Therapeutic aspiration of simple pneumothorax.

CONTRAINDICATIONS

- Coagulopathy (a relative contraindication).
- Local sepsis over intended puncture site.
- Lack of consent.

BRITISH THORACIC SOCIETY (BTS) GUIDELINES FOR MANAGING PNEUMOTHORACES

Pleural aspiration has a role in the management of pneumothoraces if certain criteria are met:

- Primary pneumothorax (no evidence of underlying lung disease):
  — if patient is not breathless or there is <2 cm rim of air on chest X-ray, observe and do not proceed to aspiration/drainage
  — if patient breathless or >2 cm rim of air on chest X-ray, then aspirate. If unsuccessful, consider repeat aspiration up to a total of 2.5 L. If an air leak persists, insert a chest drain (see Chapter 4).
- Secondary pneumothorax (known underlying lung disease):
  — if patient is not breathless, or there is <2 cm rim of air on chest X-ray, or patient is less than 50 years old, consider aspiration
  — if patient breathless or > 2 cm rim of air on chest X-ray, then insert a chest drain (see Chapter 4).

TENSION PNEUMOTHORAX – EMERGENCY MANAGEMENT

- This is a medical emergency requiring immediate recognition and treatment. If left untreated the increasing size of the tension pneumothorax compresses the mediastinum, ultimately obstructing venous return to the right heart and causing subsequent haemodynamic collapse and death.

Tip Box

Tension pneumothorax is a clinical diagnosis that **does not** require radiological confirmation – this wastes valuable time.

Tip Box

Do not waste time with local anaesthetic – warn the patient of the procedure and the importance of performing it quickly.

PROCEDURE

- Upon diagnosing a tension pneumothorax, immediately insert a large-bore cannula over the upper border of the third rib in the second anterior intercostal space, mid-clavicular line (Fig. 3.1).

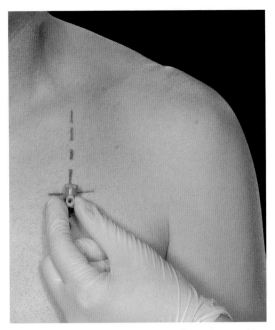

Fig. 3.1   Position for decompression of tension pneumothorax: the second intercostal space, mid-clavicular line.

- Upon removing the trocar a 'hiss' of air should be heard, signifying decompression of the tension and reversion to a simple pneumothorax.
- The purpose of needle thoracocentesis is to convert a tension pneumothorax into a simple pneumothorax. Inserting the cannula allows air to escape to atmosphere during expiration rather than accumulating and placing the intrathoracic structures under tension. Therefore formal drainage of the residual simple pneumothorax will still be required with an intercostal drain (see Chapter 4).

EQUIPMENT

- Dressing pack.
- Sterile gown, gloves and drapes.
- Chlorhexidine cleaning solution.
- Lidocaine.
- 2 × 10mL syringes.
- Orange needle.
- Green needle.

- Skin pen.
- Intravenous cannula – orange (14 G) or grey (16 G).
- Gauze.
- Three-way tap with attachable sterile tubing.
- 50 mL syringe.
- 3 × specimen pots, 1 × fluoride oxalate blood vacutainer (glucose), 1 × heparinized (arterial blood gas) syringe.
- Sterile collecting bag.
- Sterile dressing.

LOCATION OF SITE OF ASPIRATION

The aspiration of a pleural effusion versus a simple pneumothorax does not differ in technique, but the site of insertion is influenced by whether it is fluid or air being aspirated.

Tip Box

Always confirm the side to aspirate with the chest X-ray prior to starting the procedure.

PLEURAL EFFUSION

- Sit the patient upright and leaning forward over an elevated bedside table.
- The site of aspiration should be between the posterior-axillary line and the inferior angle of the scapula (Fig. 3.2).
- Alternatively chest percussion should allow detection of the effusion and the needle entered into the pleural space some 2–3 rib spaces below the highest level of the effusion.

Tip Box

Ideally, all pleural effusions should be aspirated with ultrasound guidance (see Chapter 4, National Patient Safety Agency recommendations), especially if any doubt exists about the level of the effusion detected by percussion or if the level for aspiration is close to the diaphragm (for example, in airways collapse the hemidiaphragm may be elevated). This should be used to place a mark on the skin which would safely allow an intrathoracic needle to reach the body of fluid in the pleural space. It is important that the aspiration should be performed with the patient in the same position as when the site for aspiration was marked – the fluid notoriously moves with change of position!

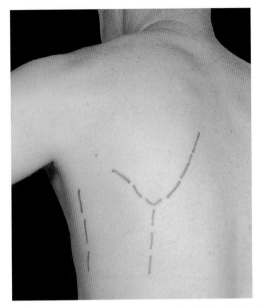

Fig. 3.2 Site for aspiration of pleural effusion: below the level of the effusion between the posterior-axillary line and the inferior angle of the scapula.

PNEUMOTHORAX

- Sit the patient upright on the bed, supported with pillows behind their head and back.
- The ideal site of aspiration is the second intercostal space in the mid-clavicular line (Fig. 3.3).

PRACTICAL PROCEDURE

PREPARATION

- Obtain consent.
- Ask a nurse to accompany you in order to open non-sterile equipment and to comfort the patient.
- Before donning the sterile gown and gloves, identify and mark the site of aspiration (described above) with a skin pen (if not already done under ultrasound guidance).
- Wash hands, wear the sterile gown and gloves and lay out sterile environment and dressing pack.

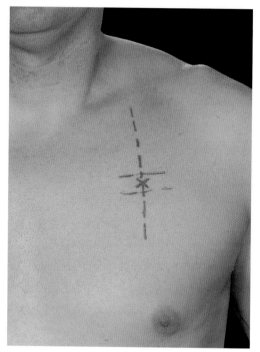

Fig. 3.3 Site for aspiration of pneumothorax: the second intercostal space, mid-clavicular line.

- Check and assemble equipment for a therapeutic pleural tap (Fig. 3.4):
  1. Connect a 50 mL syringe to a three-way tap at the port furthest from the patient.
  2. Attach sterile tubing to the port closest to the patient that will receive pleural contents via a cannula.
  3. Finally attach sterile tubing to the side-port and, if performing a therapeutic tap of a pleural effusion, connect to a sterile collecting bag.
- Fill the 10 mL syringe with lidocaine via a green needle.
- Clean the area – remember to clean outwards from the proposed site of aspiration (spirally from centre to periphery to avoid bringing dirty solution in contact with a previously cleaned area) to keep a clean field.
- Infiltrate local anaesthetic subcutaneously with an orange needle.
- Infiltrate local anaesthetic **liberally** with a green needle into deeper tissues:
  1. Advance the needle into the intercostal space just above the superior border of the lower rib (to avoid the neurovascular bundle sitting beneath the upper rib, Fig. 3.5).

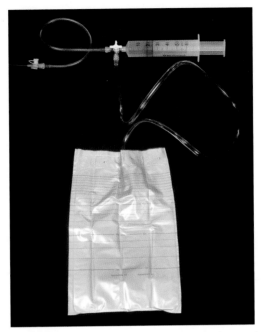

Fig. 3.4 Assembled equipment for a therapeutic pleural tap (note: the cannula is connected to the apparatus after it is in situ in the effusion).

2. Advance the needle slowly and infiltrate with anaesthetic until you aspirate air (pneumothorax) or pleural fluid. Whilst withdrawing the needle, line the track with local anaesthetic.

PROCEDURE: DIAGNOSTIC PLEURAL TAP

- Assemble a 20 mL syringe with a new green needle and simply advance (whilst continually aspirating) along the anaesthetized track. Obtain approximately 20 mL of pleural fluid.

PROCEDURE: THERAPEUTIC TAP OF A PLEURAL EFFUSION OR PNEUMOTHORAX

- Advance the cannula slowly along the anaesthetized track to the approximate depth at which air/fluid was aspirated on local anaesthetic infiltration, looking for a flashback in the case of pleural fluid.

SECTION 1 Airway and breathing

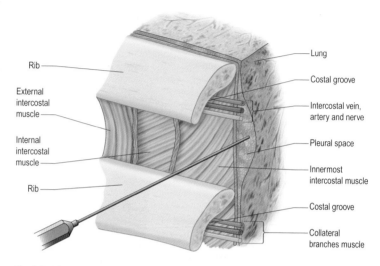

Fig. 3.5 The neurovascular bundle runs in the groove on the inferior aspect of the rib.

- Introduce the plastic cannula over its trocar into the thoracic cavity until the hub or wings of the cannula abut the skin surface.
- Whilst holding the cannula in place, remove the trocar and attach the sterile tubing connected to the three-way tap, 50 mL syringe and collecting bag.
- Turn the tap to connect the pleural space with the 50 mL syringe and aspirate 50 mL of air/fluid. Then turn the three-way tap to connect the syringe with the sterile collecting bag (the three-way tap in this position is closed to the pleural space). You will now be able to syringe out the aspirated effusion into the collecting bag, or syringe out the aspirated gas to atmosphere in the case of a pneumothorax.
- Repeat this step (counting the number of syringe-fulls of air removed if a pneumothorax) until:
  — resistance is felt
  — a dry tap is achieved
  — the patient coughs repeatedly
  — 2.5 L of air are aspirated
  — 1–1.5 L of pleural fluid are aspirated.

FINISHING OFF

- Ask the patient to breathe out whilst removing the cannula (to prevent pneumothorax) and cover the puncture site with gauze. Press on the gauze for 1–2 minutes to encourage haemostasis.

- Apply a sterile dressing.
- Document the procedure clearly in the patient's medical notes.

Tip Box

Use ultrasound guidance in the event of an unsuccessful tap to determine if the effusion is loculated. A radiologically guided drain insertion may be required in this case.

POST-PROCEDURE INVESTIGATIONS

- Biochemistry – protein, lactate dehydrogenase (LDH, standard sterile specimen container); glucose (in fluoride oxalate vacutainer).
- Microscopy, culture and sensitivity (standard sterile specimen container).
- Cytology (standard sterile specimen container).
- Fluid pH (unless debris in fluid, run sample from an arterial blood gas syringe through a blood gas analyser).
- Chest X-ray – to confirm radiological result (if therapeutic procedure) and to rule out iatrogenic pneumothorax.

Tip Box

Light's criteria provide a more sensitive tool for diagnosing an exudate. The effusion is an exudate if at least one of the following criteria are met:

1. The pleural fluid:serum protein ratio >0.5.
2. The pleural fluid:serum LDH ratio >0.6.
3. Pleural fluid LDH is greater than two-thirds the upper limit of normal value serum LDH.

COMPLICATIONS

- Bleeding.
- Infection.
- Injury to the intercostal neurovascular bundle.
- Pneumothorax.
- Re-expansion pulmonary oedema (if too much fluid is removed). Do not drain off more than 1–1.5 L of pleural fluid in one aspiration to avoid this complication. If it is known that more than 1.5 L of pleural fluid is to be drained, consider inserting an intercostal chest drain (see Chapter 4) rather than a therapeutic tap.

SECTION 1 **Airway and breathing**

SUGGESTED READING

Henry M, Arnold T, Harvey J et al 2003 BTS guidelines for the management of spontaneous pneumothorax. Thorax 58(Suppl 2): ii39.
http://thorax.bmj.com/cgi/reprint/58/suppl_2/ii39

Maskell NA, Butland RJA 2003 BTS guidelines for the investigation of a unilateral pleural effusion in adults. Thorax 58(Suppl 2): ii8.
http://thorax.bmj.com/cgi/reprint/58/suppl_2/ii8.pdf

CHEST DRAIN INSERTION AND MANAGEMENT

Hippocrates (460–377 BC) first suggested thoracocentesis by making an incision in the chest wall. However, it was not until 1850 when Henry Ingersoll Bowditch (1808–1892) and Morill Wyman (1812–1903) at the Massachusetts General Hospital demonstrated the removal of fluid from the pleural space with the use of a trocar puncturing the chest wall.

INTRODUCTION

Chest drains are used to remove fluid (including blood or pus) or air from the pleural cavity. This chapter sets out the insertion and management of chest drains in accordance with current British Thoracic Society (BTS) guidelines and National Patient Safety Agency (NPSA) recommendations.

SECTION 1 Airway and breathing

NPSA RECOMMENDATIONS

In 2008 the NPSA issued recommendations for chest drain insertion, having received reports of 12 deaths and 15 incidents of serious harm relating to this clinical procedure over a 3-year period. Common themes included inappropriate selection of the site for drain insertion, excessive insertion of the dilator giving rise to trauma, inexperienced doctors and/or poor supervision in performing the procedure, and a lack of familiarity with the Seldinger technique and/or the apparatus used. These short-comings resulted in the puncture of blood vessels with ensuing haemorrhage, or the perforation of major organs including the heart, lungs, liver and spleen.

For these reasons, the NPSA issued the following guidance relating to intercostal chest drain insertion using the modified Seldinger technique.

Drainage tubes should only be inserted by trained staff with relevant competencies and adequate supervision.

Due to the risk of damaging internal organs through poor positioning, the NPSA strongly supports the use of ultrasound when positioning a drain. The BTS also supports ultrasound-guided chest drain insertion.

Where practicable patients will be required to provide written consent prior to the procedure.

Furthermore, the NPSA re-iterated the BTS guidelines on chest drain insertion that are mentioned throughout this chapter.

INDICATIONS

- Pneumothorax:
  — in any ventilated patient
  — tension pneumothorax after initial needle relief
  — persistent or recurrent primary pneumothorax after simple aspiration
  — large secondary spontaneous pneumothorax in patients over 50 years.
- Pleural effusion (malignant or complicated parapneumonic effusion).
- Haemothorax.
- Empyema.
- Post-operative (e.g. post-cardiothoracic surgery) – this will not be covered as this should be managed by surgical teams intra-operatively.

CAUTIONS

The following differential diagnoses must be carefully evaluated with radiological guidance prior to considering chest drain insertion:

1. Pneumothorax versus bullous lung disease.
2. Pulmonary collapse versus unilateral massive pleural effusion ('white-out' on the chest X-ray).

CONTRAINDICATIONS

- Coagulopathy (recent aspirin/clopidogrel, heparin last 12 hours, international normalized ratio (INR) above 1.2, activated partial thromboplastin time ratios (APTRs) above 1.2).
- Local sepsis over drain site.
- Lack of consent.

EQUIPMENT

- Dressing pack.
- Sterile gown, gloves and drapes.
- Chlorhexidine cleaning solution.
- Lidocaine.
- 1 × 20 mL syringe.
- Orange needle.
- Green needle.
- Seldinger chest drain kit, size 10–14 F (including chest tube, guidewire with dilators, introducer needle with port for guidewire, syringe, 3-way tap).
- Connecting tubing.
- Closed drainage system (with sterile water for underwater seal).
- Gauze.
- Scalpel and blade.
- Suture (e.g. '1' silk).
- Clear sterile dressing.
- Skin pen.
- Sleek® adhesive tape.

CHOOSING THE SIZE OF CHEST DRAIN – THE GUIDELINES

An ongoing debate exists as to the optimal size of chest drain. BTS guidelines state that:

> Small bore drains are recommended as they are more comfortable than larger bore tubes, but there is no evidence that either is therapeutically superior.

10–14 F catheters are commonly used sizes of drain by physicians, and can be inserted simply using the Seldinger technique. The NPSA estimates that approximately 85–90% of chest drains inserted in clinical practice are done so by the modified Seldinger technique.

The only exception to this recommendation applies to the drainage of acute haemothorax, in which large-bore drains (inserted by blunt dissection, 28–30 F minimum) are advised in order to monitor further blood loss. Given that this situation

SECTION 1 **Airway and breathing**

arises in the context of trauma (managed by the trauma team) rather than the other indications for chest drains (managed by general physicians), blunt dissection will not be covered in this review. Blunt dissection is, however, covered in Chapter 5.

Tip Box: Pre-Medication

- Pre-medication with either an intravenous benzodiazepine (immediately pre-procedure) *or* intramuscular opioid agent (1 hour pre-procedure) is recommended as routine unless there is potential for a significant complication (for example, respiratory depression in those with chronic obstructive airways disease).
- It is prudent to monitor the patient closely having administered the pre-medication, and have the appropriate antidote to hand in the event of respiratory depression (flumazenil and naloxone for benzodiazepines and opiates, respectively).

POSITION FOR DRAIN INSERTION

- The patient should be positioned sitting up on the bed and slightly rotated, exposing the axilla with the ipsilateral arm placed behind their head.
- Alternatively, the patient could sit upright and lean on pillows placed on an elevated bedside table.

SITE OF DRAIN INSERTION

The insertion of a chest drain for drainage of a pleural effusion versus a pneumothorax does not differ in technique, but in terms of site of insertion:

- For an effusion the drain should be inserted in the mid-axillary line below the level of the fluid.
- For a pneumothorax, the drain should be inserted in the mid-axillary line of the 'safe triangle' as per BTS guidelines (Fig. 4.1).

The apex of the safe triangle is just below the axilla, with its borders being the anterior border of the latissimus dorsi muscle, the lateral border of the pectoralis major muscle, and a line extending from the level of the nipple.

Prior to procedure always confirm the side for drain insertion with the chest X-ray. (BTS guidelines).

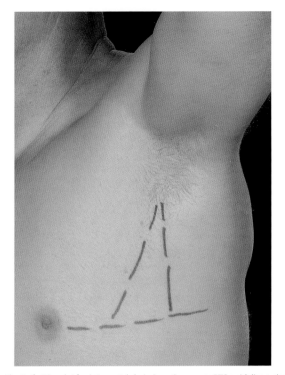

Fig. 4.1 The 'safe triangle' for intercostal drain insertion as per BTS guidelines: the apex just below the axilla, and the borders being the anterior border of latissimus dorsi, the lateral border of pectoralis major and a line extending from the level of the nipple.

PRACTICAL PROCEDURE

- Obtain consent.
- Ask a nurse to accompany you in order to open non-sterile equipment and to comfort the patient.
- Before donning the sterile gown and gloves, mark the site of drain insertion with a skin pen.
- Wash hands, wear the sterile gown and gloves and lay out sterile environment and dressing pack.
- Check and assemble equipment – fill the underwater seal bottles with sterile water to the marked level, and attach to the connecting tube. Fill the 10 mL syringe with lidocaine via a green needle (your assistant offering the lidocaine to the needle).

SECTION 1 **Airway and breathing**

- Clean the area – remember to clean outwards from the proposed site of insertion (spirally from centre to periphery to avoid bringing dirty solution in contact with a previously cleaned area) to keep a clean field.
- Infiltrate local anaesthetic subcutaneously with an orange needle.
- Infiltrate local anaesthetic with a green needle into deeper tissues:
  — advance the needle vertically just above the superior border of the rib (to avoid the neurovascular bundle, see Fig. 3.5)
  — advance the needle slowly and infiltrate with anaesthetic until you aspirate air (pneumothorax) or pleural fluid. Whilst withdrawing the needle, line the track **liberally** with local anaesthetic (Fig. 4.2).

Tip Box

A chest drain should not be inserted without further image guidance if free air or fluid cannot be aspirated with a needle at the time of anaesthesia. (BTS guidelines)

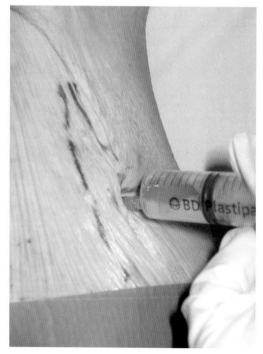

Fig. 4.2   Line the track with local anaesthetic.

- Attach the 5 mL syringe to the introducer needle and insert vertically along the anaesthetized track whilst aspirating.
  — Insert the needle bevel up for pneumothoraces, bevel down for effusions.
- Having reached the pleural cavity, hold the needle still with your non-dominant hand and remove the syringe with the other. Now pass the guidewire down the introducer needle.
- Ensuring that you do not lose sight of the guidewire at any time, remove the needle over the guidewire (Fig. 4.3).
- Make a small incision (approximately 0.5 cm) in the skin immediately adjacent to the guidewire to enlarge the guidewire's percutaneous passage.
- Pass the dilator over the guidewire, ensuring that the guidewire appears from the other end of the dilator before it touches the skin (Fig. 4.4).

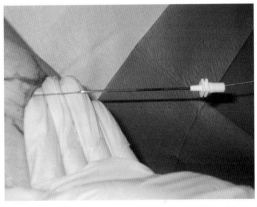

Fig. 4.3 Remove the needle over the guidewire without losing sight of the guidewire.

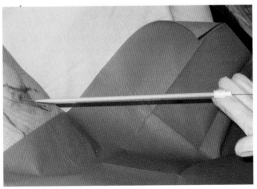

Fig. 4.4 Ensure the guidewire appears from the other end of the dilator before it touches the skin.

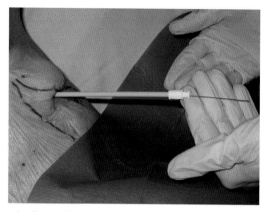

Fig. 4.5 Pass the dilator without substantial force using a rotating motion.

- Whilst holding the guidewire at its tip, insert the dilator through the skin into the pleural cavity using a rotating motion (Fig. 4.5).
    — **Do not** advance the dilator further than the distance that was required to pass the needle in order to aspirate the contents of the pleural cavity at the time of local anaesthetic administration (see NPSA recommendations above).

Tip Box

Chest drain insertion should be performed without substantial force. (BTS guidelines).

- Whilst holding the guidewire *at all times*, remove the dilator over the guidewire and cover the puncture site with gauze.
- Estimate the length of tube to be inserted into the pleural cavity by checking the length of tube against the patient's chest. The tip should be sited at the apex in the case of a pneumothorax, and aimed basally for pleural fluid.
- Pass the drain over the guidewire, ensuring that the guidewire appears from the other end of the drain before it touches the skin.
- Whilst holding the guidewire at its tip, insert the chest drain through the skin.
- If draining a pneumothorax, ask the patient to hold their breath. Quickly remove the guidewire and attach the 3-way tap in the 'closed' position (Fig. 4.6).
- Secure the drain in position with a single suture.

    — Insert a suture next to the drain with equidistant lengths of suture material either side.
    — Using the two lengths of suture material, wrap them tightly around the drain in a 'plaiting' fashion. Having plaited the suture material for a reasonable length (at least five plaits) tie the sutures off (Fig. 4.7).

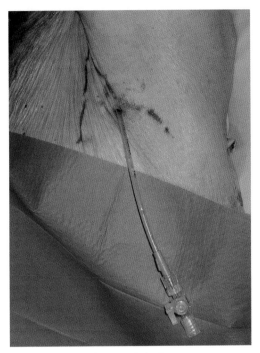

Fig. 4.6   Having inserted the chest drain, attach the 3-way tap.

Tip Box

'Purse string' sutures must not be used, as they convert a linear wound into a circular one that is painful for the patient and may leave an unsightly scar. (BTS guidelines).

— Overlay an 'omental tag' of tape on the plaiting approximately 2 cm from the skin surface (Fig. 4.8). This further secures the drain while allowing the tube to lie away from the thoracic wall.

— Apply a transparent dressing to the insertion site in order to inspect for leakage or infection. DO NOT apply large amounts of gauze or dressing material or tape to the insertion site – this will hide any signs of local sepsis or leakage.

• Connect the 3-way tap to the tubing of the chest drain bottle and open the tap. Fluid/bubbling should now be observed.

• Document the procedure clearly in the medical notes.

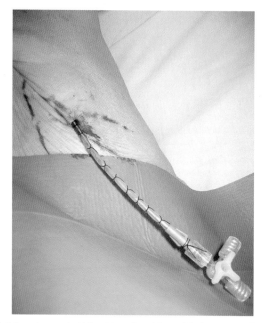

Fig. 4.7 Plait the suture material for at least five plaits and tie the sutures off.

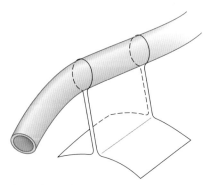

Fig. 4.8 An 'omental tag' of tape. (Reproduced from Laws D, Neville E, Duffy J (2003) BTS guidelines for the insertion of a chest drain. Thorax 58:ii53.)

POST-PROCEDURE INVESTIGATIONS

- Chest X-ray – to confirm drain position and therapeutic result.
- If an effusion, send for biochemistry, microscopy, culture and sensitivity, cytology and fluid pH (as described previously, see Chapter 3).

POST-PROCEDURE CARE

- Prescribe oral analgesia.
- In order to avoid the rare complication of re-expansion pulmonary oedema, do not drain off more than 2 L of pleural fluid in 24 hours (e.g. 1 L mane, 1 L nocte).
- The patient should be admitted to a ward where the nursing staff are trained to manage chest drains.
- For the underwater seal, it is imperative that the bottle is kept below the level of the insertion site **at all times** (to prevent passage of the drainage bottle contents into the pleural cavity). The bottle must also be kept upright, and adequate sterile water should be present in order to submerge the end of the tube.
- Record regularly the amount of drainage/bubbling and the presence of respiratory swing on a dedicated chest drain chart.

COMPLICATIONS

- Pain.
- Bleeding.
- Infection.
- Injury to the intercostal neurovascular bundle.
- Injury to intrathoracic structures and lung parenchyma.
- Pneumothorax.
- Surgical emphysema.
- Re-expansion pulmonary oedema.

SUGGESTED READING

Henry M, Arnold T, Harvey J et al (2003) BTS guidelines for the management of spontaneous pneumothorax. Thorax 58(Suppl 2): ii39.
http://thorax.bmj.com/cgi/reprint/58/suppl_2/ii39

Laws D, Neville E, Duffy J (2003) BTS guidelines for the insertion of a chest drain. Thorax 58(Suppl 2): ii53.
http://thorax.bmj.com/cgi/reprint/58/suppl_2/ii53

NPSA (2008) Risks of chest drain insertion.
http://www.npsa.nhs.uk/patientsafety/alerts-and-directives/rapidrr/risks-of-chest-drain-insertion/

PERCUTANEOUS PLEURAL BIOPSY

Pleural biopsy, originally an open technique, has been more commonly performed blindly ever since Abrams' description using a specialized needle in 1958. Prior to Abrams' development, the original technique used a Franklin modification of the Vim-Silverman needle, which was used for renal biopsy. Despite Cope also describing a novel needle for pleural biopsy in 1958, the Abrams' needle remains the most popular apparatus. Recently there has been interest in ultrasound-guided biopsies with both modified Abrams' needles and needles that only require a single pass for multiple biopsies.

Tip Box

Image guided cutting needle biopsies have a higher yield for malignancy than standard Abrams' needle pleural biopsy.
(British Thoracic Society guidelines)

INTRODUCTION

Percutaneous pleural biopsy is occasionally performed when other means for reaching a diagnosis of an exudative pleural effusion have not been successful. Pleural aspirate examination coupled with cross-sectional imaging and cytology obtained at bronchoscopy will usually provide sufficient data to make a diagnosis. Percutaneous pleural biopsy is, however, recommended when standard cytology is non-diagnostic. The procedure is particularly useful when granulomatous or malignant disease of the pleura is suspected.

CONTRAINDICATIONS

- Coagulopathy.
- Local sepsis over biopsy site.
- Lack of consent.

EQUIPMENT

- Dressing pack.
- Sterile gown, gloves and drapes.
- Chlorhexidine cleaning solution.
- Lidocaine.
- 1 × 10 mL syringe.
- 1 × 20 mL syringe.
- Orange needle.
- Green needle.
- Skin pen.
- Gauze.
- Scalpel.
- Clamped forceps (one for blunt dissection and one for chest drain insertion if required).
- If a chest drain is to be inserted post-biopsy: large-bore chest drain kit, connecting tubing, closed drainage system (with sterile water for underwater seal), suture (e.g. '1' silk).
- Sterile dressing.
- 3 sterile specimen pots (for biochemistry, microscopy culture and sensitivity, cytology) and specimen pots for histology (containing formaldehyde solution).
- Abrams' needle (Fig. 5.1).

Tip Box

Practice 'playing' with the Abrams' needle so that you are completely familiar with its workings.

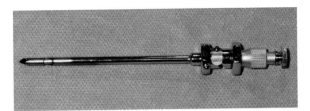

Fig. 5.1 The assembled Abrams' needle.

THE ABRAMS' NEEDLE

The Abrams' needle consists of three separate components (Fig. 5.2):

- An outer cannula with a trocar point. The cutting window (Fig. 5.3) is closed by turning the inner tube, thus severing pleural tissue against the sharp cutting edge and catching it in the inner tube.
- The catch on the inner cannula runs in the groove on the outer cannula (Fig. 5.4), thus securing the cutting window in either the open or closed position.
- The innermost tube, a blunt obturator.

Tip Box: Pre-Medication
- Pre-medication with either an intravenous benzodiazepine (immediately pre-procedure) *or* intramuscular opioid agent (1 hour pre-procedure) is recommended as routine unless a contraindication to its use exists.
  — Care should be taken to ensure that the respiratory centre depressant side-effect of sedatives does not complicate the already compromised ventilatory function of patients with conditions such as chronic obstructive pulmonary disease.
  — It is therefore prudent to monitor the patient closely having administered the pre-medication, and have the appropriate antidote to hand in the event of respiratory depression (flumazenil and naloxone for benzodiazepines and opiates, respectively).

SITE OF BIOPSY

- The patient should sit upright and lean on pillows placed on an elevated bedside table.
- The biopsy should be taken in the mid-axillary line below the level of the fluid.
- **Always confirm the side for biopsy with the chest X-ray pre-procedure.**

SECTION 1 **Airway and breathing**

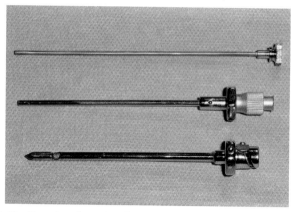

Fig. 5.2 The Abrams' needle consists of three separate components.

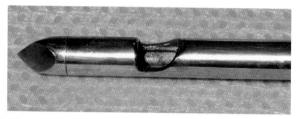

Fig. 5.3 The cutting window severs pleural tissue against the cutting edge.

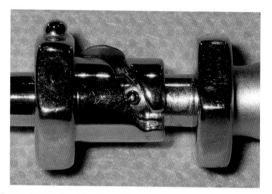

Fig. 5.4 The mechanism by which the cutting window is opened and closed: the catch on the inner cannula runs in the groove on the outer cannula.

PRACTICAL PROCEDURE

- Obtain consent.
- Ask a nurse to accompany you in order to open non-sterile equipment and to comfort the patient.
- Before donning the sterile gown and gloves, mark the site of drain insertion with a skin pen.
- Wash hands, wear the sterile gown and gloves and lay out sterile environment and dressing pack.
- Fill the 10 mL syringe with lidocaine via a green needle.
- Clean the area – remember to clean outwards from the proposed site of insertion (spirally from centre to periphery to avoid bringing dirty solution in contact with a previously cleaned area) to keep a clean field.
- Infiltrate local anaesthetic subcutaneously with orange needle.
- Infiltrate local anaesthetic with a green needle into deeper tissues:
  — advance the needle just above the superior border of the rib thus avoiding the neurovascular bundle
  — advance the needle slowly and infiltrate with anaesthetic until you aspirate pleural fluid. Whilst withdrawing the needle, line the track *liberally* with local anaesthetic.
- Attach the 20 mL syringe to a green needle, and insert the needle along the anaesthetized track whilst aspirating. Aspirate 20 mL of pleural fluid for diagnostic investigations (outlined below).
- Make a horizontal 2 cm incision in the anaesthetized skin.
- Use the clamped forceps to blunt dissect down through the subcutaneous fat and intercostal muscles to the pleural space, at which point pleural fluid will appear from the dissected track. Blunt dissection (the separation of tissue without incision) is performed by carefully but forcibly inserting the closed forceps into the tissue and subsequently opening them, thus pushing the tissue layers apart (Fig. 5.5). When blunt dissecting skeletal muscle, part the muscle layers in line with the muscle striae. A track should be made large enough to accommodate your finger.
- Insert the Abrams' needle with the outer window open and pointing at 9 o'clock. Push the needle laterally against the chest wall and then slowly pull the needle backwards so that the outer window catches against the pleura.
- Whilst applying this tension against the pleura, rotate the inner needle in order to close the window and lock it in place. Now pull the entire apparatus back, effectively tearing the pleura caught within the needle.
- Place the sample in formaldehyde-containing specimen pots. Macroscopically, pleura appears pearl-like in colour.
- '*When using an Abrams' needle, at least four biopsy specimens should be taken from one site*' (British Thoracic Society guidelines). Repeat the biopsies at 6 and 3 o'clock (not at 12 o'clock – this risks injury to the neurovascular bundle above).
- Having completed the biopsies, a chest drain may be inserted directly down the track already created. Grasp the tip of the chest drain with clamped forceps and, placing

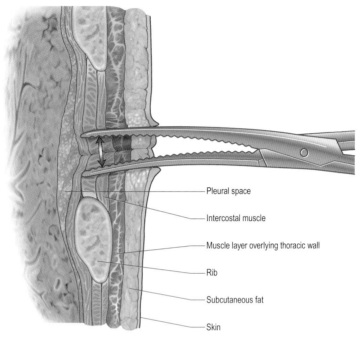

Pleural space

Intercostal muscle

Muscle layer overlying thoracic wall

Rib

Subcutaneous fat

Skin

Fig. 5.5 Blunt dissection.

your finger superiorly in the track to guard against injury to the neurovascular bundle above, introduce the tip of the drain into the pleural cavity (Fig. 5.6).

- Once in the pleural cavity, open and remove the clamped forceps and slide the required length of chest drain into the pleural space. Connect to a closed underwater drainage system as described in Chapter 4.
- Document the procedure clearly in the medical notes.

POST-PROCEDURE INVESTIGATIONS

- Chest X-ray – to rule out pneumothorax.
- Send effusion for biochemistry, microscopy, culture and sensitivity, cytology and fluid pH (see Chapter 3).
- Send pleural tissue for histology, AAFB smear and culture.

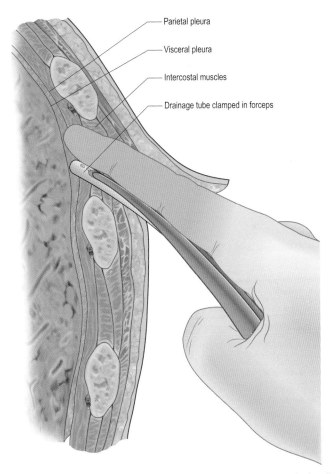

Fig. 5.6 Introducing a chest drain with forceps whilst shielding the neurovascular bundle with your finger.

POST-PROCEDURE CARE

- Prescribe oral analgesia.

CAUTIONS

Patients with proven or suspected mesothelioma should receive prophylactic radiotherapy to the site of biopsy or chest drain insertion. (BTS guidelines).

Up to 40% of patients with mesothelioma may develop seeding at the site of pleural biopsy or chest drain insertion. Local radiotherapy to the site is indicated within 1 month in all patients who have undergone such procedures in whom the final diagnosis is mesothelioma.

COMPLICATIONS

- Pain.
- Haemothorax.
- Haematoma.
- Infection.
- Injury to the intercostal neurovascular bundle.
- Pneumothorax.

SUGGESTED READING

Chakrabarti B, Ryland I, Sheard J et al (2006) The role of Abrams percutaneous pleural biopsy in the investigation of exudative pleural effusions. Chest 129(6): 1549.

http://www.chestjournal.org/content/129/6/1549.full.pdf

Antunes G, Neville E, Duffy J, Ali N (2003) BTS guidelines for the management of malignant pleural effusions. Thorax 58(Suppl 2): ii29.

http://thorax.bmj.com/cgi/reprint/58/suppl_2/ii29.pdf

VENEPUNCTURE (PERIPHERAL AND FEMORAL)

Venesection is probably the oldest surgical intervention. It was used therapeutically by Hippocrates (460–377 BC), while Aulus Cornelius Celsus (25 BC–AD 50) gave it a scientific context and described the technique in *De Re Medicina*. It became a universal remedy in virtually all cultures. It had spectacular results in those with pulmonary oedema secondary to rheumatic heart disease but was less successful in those with asthma, convulsions, etc., where it was equally applied and consequently was the source of controversy as a universal remedy. In Graeco-Arabic medicine (Unani) it was thought to let out putrid humours. This concept was later supplemented by the practice of blood fortification by the administration of iron-containing substances. Such practice persisted well into the 19th century in the western world. Today venesection is largely for investigative rather than therapeutic purposes.

INTRODUCTION

Phlebotomy or venepuncture is a basic clinical skill that is routinely practised by a number of health professionals. Peripheral venepuncture should be performed efficiently with minimal discomfort to the patient. Occasionally peripheral venepuncture may be difficult or contraindicated and femoral venepuncture is indicated.

SECTION 2   Circulation

INDICATIONS

- Routine blood investigations: haematology; biochemistry; immunology.
- Transfusion samples: group and cross-match/group and save.
- Toxicology samples: therapeutic drug monitoring (e.g. gentamicin, vancomycin, phenytoin levels); assays in overdose (e.g. paracetamol).
- Microbiology investigations: blood cultures (covered in a later chapter); serology.

CONTRAINDICATIONS

- Local infection.
- Superficial or deep venous thrombosis.
- Ipsilateral mastectomy, (i.e. a limb with impaired lymphatic drainage).
- Ipsilateral hemiparesis or contractures.
- Ipsilateral arterio-venous fistula.
- Lack of consent.

PERIPHERAL VENEPUNCTURE EQUIPMENT

- Vacutainer® needle or Monovette® needle.
- Vacutainer® barrel or Monovette® attachment.
- Sterile alcohol swabs.
- Blood bottles (Fig. 6.1).
- Gloves.

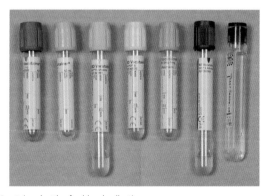

Fig. 6.1 Vacutainer bottles for blood collection.

- Cotton wool balls.
- Plaster.
- Tourniquet.

PRACTICAL PROCEDURE

- Explain the procedure to the patient and gain consent.
- Check the paper seal is intact on the Vacutainer needle to ensure sterility (Fig. 6.2).
- Break the paper seal and twist the Vacutainer needle into the barrel.
- Place the arm on a comfortable surface such as a pillow.
- Place tourniquet on the upper arm sufficiently tight to distend veins but not occlude the artery (check the pulse is palpable below the tourniquet).
- Look and feel for a vein, noting the size and direction of the vein (Fig. 6.3). Start in the antecubital fossa and work your way down the arm. Aim to select a vein that has not been used recently for venepuncture, is easily located, feels bouncy and refills quickly when pressure is applied.

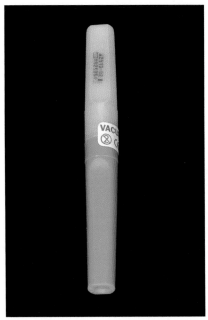

Fig. 6.2   Check the paper seal is intact on the Vacutainer needle.

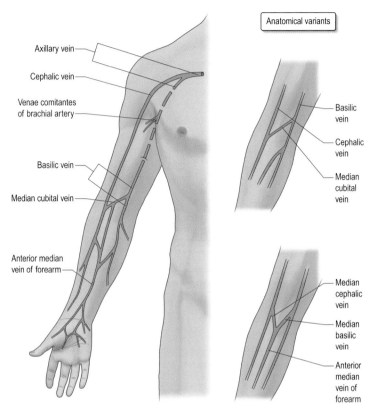

Fig. 6.3 Anatomy of the venous system of the forearm.

Tip Box

If there are unsuitable or difficult to locate veins on one arm:

- Try looking in the other arm.
- Ask the patient to open and close their fist, thereby increasing venous return against the tourniquet and distending the veins.
- Tapping the veins causes venodilatation and might aid finding a suitable site.
- Hang the arm off the side of the bed for a few minutes below the level of the heart.
- Immerse the patient's arm in warm water or a warm towel in order to dilate the veins.

- If this fails, a GTN patch applied topically will also promote local venodilatation.
- Certain groups of patients who have had previous access difficulties may be able to guide you given their previous hospital experiences, e.g. patients with chronic co-morbidities such as chronic renal failure or intravenous drug users.

- Wash your hands and wear gloves.
- Clean the area of skin with sterile alcohol swabs and allow to dry.

Tip Box

If taking a sample for blood alcohol concentrations, avoid cleaning with isopropyl alcohol and use soap and water. Although there is little chance of altering blood alcohol concentrations, samples are often taken in a law enforcement context.

- Remove sheath from the Vacutainer needle.
- Stretch the skin a few centimetres above (or below) the area of presumed vene-puncture with the thumb of your non-dominant hand so that needle insertion is not deviated by the elasticity of the skin.
- Warn the patient of a sharp scratch.
- Gently insert the needle into the vein at a 30–45 degree angle with the bevel facing upwards.

Tip Box

When placing the vacutainer needle into the vein don't have the blood bottle pre-attached to the barrel. The vacuum in the blood bottle will collapse the vein on entry.

- Holding the Vacutainer steady with your hand resting stable against the patient's arm, insert the blood bottles into the Vacutainer barrel and allow the vacuum in the bottles to fill them up. Try to fill bottles to the indicated mark; laboratories often reject small samples.
- When the flow of blood into the bottle stops, remove the bottle whilst holding the barrel steady.

- Remove the tourniquet.
- Remove the needle and immediately place the cotton wool over the venepuncture site, pressing firmly for 2 minutes.

Tip Box

Do not flex the arm after peripheral venepuncture as this predisposes to haematoma formation.

- Gently mix the blood bottle contents by inverting them upside down a few times.
- Having asked the patient if they have a plaster allergy, place a plaster over the venepuncture site.

Tip Box

For patients with veins that are small, fragile or in a position that is difficult to access with a Vacutainer, a 'butterfly needle' (Fig. 6.4) may be useful. They may also be useful in patients with spasticity (secondary to hemiparesis or contractures). Attach a Vacutainer set (with a different Vacutainer needle attachment for the barrel) or a 10 mL syringe to the distal end of the butterfly needle flexible tubing. Holding the pliable butterfly wings insert the needle into the vein, approaching at a shallow (approximately 20 degree) angle. A small flashback of blood will be seen in the tubing, indicating that the butterfly needle is in the vein and that blood may now be drawn off.

Tip Box

When using a small-gauge butterfly needle take care not to aspirate too quickly as this can result in haemolysis of the sample.

FEMORAL VENEPUNCTURE EQUIPMENT

- Green needle.
- 20 mL syringe.
- Chlorhexidine cleaning solution.
- Blood bottles.
- Gloves.
- Cotton wool balls.
- Plaster.
- Sterile gauze.

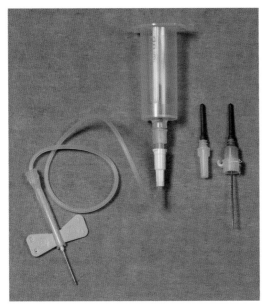

Fig. 6.4   Butterfly needle.

PRACTICAL PROCEDURE

- Explain the procedure to the patient and gain consent.
- Ensure you have the correct blood bottles and equipment.
- Assemble the needle to the syringe.
- Ensure the patient is lying flat and comfortably on a bed.
- Wash hands and wear gloves.
- Locate the femoral pulse in the groin (mid way between the symphysis pubis and anterior iliac tuberosity pushing the artery against the ischium). The femoral artery lies about one finger's breath lateral to the femoral vein (Fig. 6.5).
- Clean the skin with chlorhexidine solution and allow to dry.
- Warn the patient of a sharp scratch.
- While feeling the femoral pulse with your non-dominant hand insert the needle at a 90 degree angle (i.e. vertically) 2 cm medial to the femoral arterial pulse with the bevel facing upwards.
- The femoral vein is usually punctured at a depth of 2–4 cm, but this varies enormously with adiposity.
- When you have flashback into the needle, pull back the syringe plunger with your dominant hand until you have collected the required volume of blood.

Tip Box

If while performing femoral vein puncture you accidentally puncture the femoral artery continue to take blood anyway, and upon removing the needle apply firm pressure with a cotton wool ball for at least 5 minutes.

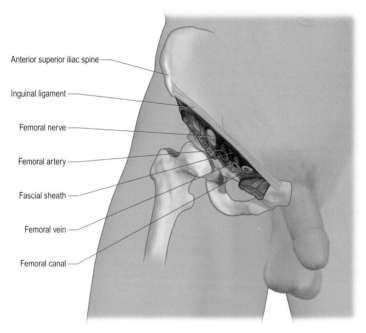

Anterior superior iliac spine

Inguinal ligament

Femoral nerve

Femoral artery

Fascial sheath

Femoral vein

Femoral canal

Fig. 6.5   The femoral vein lies medial to the femoral artery (remember the acronym NAVY from lateral to medial: Nerve, Artery, Vein, Y-fronts!).

- If there is no blood flashback into the needle, you may have gone too deeply. Gently maintain suction and withdraw the needle slowly until blood flashes back. If there is still no flashback, withdraw the needle further (but not out of the skin) and aim slightly closer to the arterial pulsation. Subsequently re-advance while maintaining suction on the syringe plunger.

Tip Box

Should the patient experience pain radiating down the leg during femoral venepuncture, this may indicate the needle hitting the femoral nerve and you are too lateral. Remove the needle and re-palpate the femoral artery, aiming medially to this landmark.

- Once blood has been obtained, remove the needle and immediately compress the venepuncture site for 3 minutes with cotton wool.
- Place a plaster over the venepuncture site

POST-PROCEDURE INVESTIGATIONS

- Label bottles.
- Ensure the blood forms are filled out correctly including the details needed for cross-match and group and save samples.
- If the blood sample is known to be 'high risk' (suspected or known HIV, AIDS, hepatitis or tropical disease and high-risk groups) attach a Bio Hazard sticker to the sample and sample bag and request form.

COMPLICATIONS

- Failed peripheral venepuncture:
  — gain consent to try an alternative vein, e.g. other antecubital fossa, back of hand, feet
  — if other sites fail and there is no contraindication, perform femoral venepuncture
  — ask someone more experienced. Don't persist more than three times.
- Local bruising.
- Arterial puncture.
- Superficial vein thrombosis.
- Deep vein thrombosis.
- Erythema and cellulitis at puncture site.
- Haemorrhage at venepuncture site.
- Vasovagal attacks.

SECTION 2 **Circulation**

BLOOD CULTURES

Following on from Louis Pasteur's (1822–1895) germ theory it was inevitable that attempts would be made to grow and isolate germs present on or within the body. Pasteur prepared a sterilized culture medium in 1861 from sugar, yeast and ammonium tartrate dissolved in water. However, it was Friedrich August Johannes Löffler (1852–1915) in 1887 who set the scene for further developments, devising horse serum, meat broth and dextrose-based 'Löffler's' medium for cultivation and separation of corynebacteria from other organisms. The German bacteriologist Julius Richard Petri (1852–1921) introduced plates, 'Petri' dishes, for bacterial culture in 1887. The process of blood acquisition, modifying culture medium contents, culturing and sub-culturing bacteria for identification was pioneered in the early 20th century. Determination of sensitivity patterns followed with the discovery of antibiotics.

INTRODUCTION

Blood cultures are an essential part of a septic screen. Growth and identification of an organism in blood culture allows the physician to consider initial antibiotic therapy which might be modified once antibiotic sensitivities of the organism are determined. In general it takes about 48 hours for culture and organism identification and a further 24 hours to determine antibiotic sensitivities. Most patients with suspected infection will already be on antibiotics, the results of cultures confirming or refuting the appropriateness of the empirical treatment. The importance of blood culture results cannot be overestimated, and therefore meticulous preparation is required to avoid false positives with sufficient blood to avoid false negatives.

INDICATIONS

- Pyrexia.
- As part of a septic screen.

SAMPLING CONTRAINDICATED

- Lack of consent.
- Sampling from the following sites to avoid false positive results:
  — Cellulitis around intended venepuncture site.
  — Superficial or deep venous thrombosis.
  — In situ peripheral cannula.
- Sampling from the following sites to prevent local complications:
  — Ipsilateral mastectomy, i.e. a limb with impaired lymphatic drainage.
  — Ipsilateral arterio-venous fistula.

EQUIPMENT

- 10 mL syringe.
- 3 × sterile alcohol swabs.
- 2 × green needles.
- Blood culture bottles (Fig. 7.1).

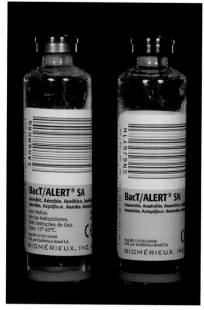

Fig. 7.1 Aerobic and anaerobic blood culture bottles. Always label the date and time of the sample.

- Tourniquet.
- Gloves.
- Cotton wool balls.
- Plaster.

PRACTICAL PROCEDURE

- Explain procedure to patient and obtain consent.
- Place the arm on a comfortable surface such as a pillow.
- Place tourniquet on the upper arm to distend veins.
- Look and feel for a vein, noting the size and direction of the vein. Start in the antecubital fossa and work your way down the arm.
- Aim to select a vein that has not recently been used for venepuncture, is easily located, feels bouncy and refills quickly when pressure is applied.
- Wash your hands and wear gloves.
- Clean the area of skin extensively with sterile alcohol swabs and allow to dry.
- Attach the green needle to the 10 mL syringe.
- Stretch the skin taut a few centimetres above or below the area of presumed venepuncture.
- Warn the patient of a sharp scratch.
- Gently insert the needle into the vein at a 30–45 degree angle with the bevel facing upwards.
- Aspirate 10 mL of blood from the patient. Alternatively use the Vacutainer system (see Chapter 6), ensuring approximately 5 mL blood is inoculated in each culture bottle.
- Remove the tourniquet.
- Remove the needle and immediately place the cotton wool over the venepuncture site and press firmly for 2 minutes.
- Place a plaster over the venepuncture site.
- Remove the tops from the blood culture bottles and place on a flat surface.
- Swab the tops of the culture bottles with sterile alcohol swabs.
- Using a new green needle inoculate each culture bottle with the volume of blood indicated on the bottles. Inoculate the aerobic bottle (blue top) first.

POST-PROCEDURE INVESTIGATIONS

- Label the bottles (including patient details and sample details, i.e. date and time of culture) and send to the microbiology laboratory.
- Ensure to indicate on the microbiology form where the cultures are taken from, i.e. peripheral blood cultures, or blood cultures taken from a line (state site).

Tip Box

If the patient has a central line (either long- or short-term), obtain blood for cultures from the line using an aseptic technique. Remember to remove the first 10 mL of blood and discard prior to obtaining the sample itself. Flush the line with 10 mL of normal saline post-aspiration to ensure line patency. Note there is still some possibility of picking up contaminants from the line, which result in false positives. Therefore, peripheral blood cultures should always be taken concurrently when taking cultures from an indwelling venous line.

Tip Box

Always fill the two culture bottles (one for aerobic, another for anaerobic organisms; laboratories may have special bottles available for fungal culture) with the volume of blood required. Modern blood culture methodology relies on automated quantitative detection of carbon dioxide derived from micro-organism metabolism. Insufficient blood will produce less carbon dioxide, which might produce a false–negative result. The chances of obtaining a true–positive blood culture result while reducing the risk of contaminants is also improved by taking two sets of cultures from different sites in close temporal proximity.

PERIPHERAL VENOUS CANNULATION

Drugs, namely opium and *Crocus metallorum*, were first administered intravenously to dogs by Sir Christopher Wren (1632–1723) in 1656 by use of a quill and bladder. This was first performed in humans by Johann Daniel Major (1634–1693) in 1662. Intravenous indwelling cannulae were popularized in the 19th and 20th centuries and were entirely metallic until the 1960s, which saw the introduction of plastic cannulae inserted both through and over metal stylets.

INTRODUCTION

Peripheral venous cannulation is a basic skill routinely required of doctors on a daily basis, and as such is important to master above virtually any other skill. Try to practise firstly on dummy models and then on patients before you qualify. This should minimize the discomfort for patients and increase your chances of success.

INDICATIONS

- Intravenous fluids.
- Intravenous medication.
- Intravenous electrolyte correction.

Tip Box

If blood is required for sampling in addition to intravenous access, withdraw blood from the newly sited cannula with a sterile syringe prior to flushing to avoid the need for a separate puncture.

CONTRAINDICATIONS

- Lack of consent.
- Cellulitis over the area of presumed cannula insertion.
- Superficial or deep venous thrombosis.
- Ipsilateral mastectomy, i.e. a limb with impaired lymphatic drainage.
- Ipsilateral hemiparesis or contractures.
- Ipsilateral arterio-venous fistula (or potential site of arterio-venous fistula formation in pre-dialysis patients).

EQUIPMENT

- Sterile alcohol swabs.
- Tourniquet.
- Cannula (see Fig. 8.1 and Table 8.1 for sizes/functions).

Tip Box

A cannula with a smaller lumen will permit better venous flow around the cannula, thus improving haemodilution of the administered drug. Larger-gauge cannulae can also cause venous occlusion and/or intimal damage. Therefore, when intravenous access is required for routine intravenous fluids or medications, insert smaller-gauge cannulae where possible.

- Three-way tap.
- Gloves.
- Gauze.
- 10 mL normal saline.
- 10 mL syringe.
- Cannula dressing.

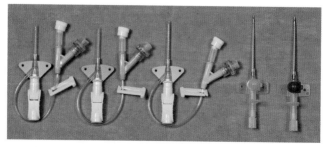

Fig. 8.1 Different-sized cannulae have different indications (see Table 8.1).

TABLE 8.1 Cannula sizes and suitable uses

Colour	Size (gauge)	Flow rate (mL/min)	Use
Blue	22	36	Patients with small veins (such as the elderly)
Pink	20	61	For routine i.v. fluids and medications
Green	18	90	
White	17	140	Large-bore access for rapid volume replacement (e.g. acute haemorrhage) and peripheral administration of potentially phlebotoxic drugs (e.g. amiodarone)
Grey	16	200	
Brown	14	300	

PRACTICAL PROCEDURE

- Explain the procedure to the patient and obtain consent.
- Fill 10 mL of normal saline into the syringe.
- Place the arm on a comfortable surface such as a pillow.
- Place tourniquet on the upper arm sufficiently tight to distend veins but not occlude the artery (check the pulse is palpable below the tourniquet).
- Look and feel for a vein, noting the size and direction of the vein (see Fig. 6.3). Start distally and work proximally towards the antecubital fossa. Conversely, if large-bore access is required (especially in cases of haemodynamic instability), aim for a large vein in the antecubital fossa.

Tip Box

It is best to avoid placing the cannula at a 'positional' site (e.g. at a joint) in patients who are confused or unable to keep the limb still, as lumen patency and thus infusion flow through the cannula is compromised by patient movement in that region.

- Wash your hands and wear gloves.
- Swab the skin overlying the target vein and allow to dry.

Tip Box

For cannulae 16 G or larger local anaesthetic should be administered to the puncture site (it is a lot easier to be allowed a second go if the first attempt was painless!). Local anaesthetic cream can be applied under an occlusive dressing or intradermal lidocaine injected over the proposed venepuncture site. Wait for a few minutes after anaesthetic application then proceed.

- Stretch the skin taut above or below the presumed cannula site to render the vein immobile.
- Warn the patient of a sharp scratch.
- Gently insert the cannula at a 20–30 degree angle into the vein with the bevel facing upwards and in the direction of venous return (Fig. 8.2).
- You may feel a give as you enter the vein. Look for a flashbak of blood into the cannula (Fig. 8.3).
- With your non-dominant hand gently withdraw the stylet 1 mm or so and watch for blood flow into the cannula (indicating it is positioned in the lumen of the vein (Fig. 8.4A). Then slide the cannula into the vein over the needle (Fig. 8.4B).

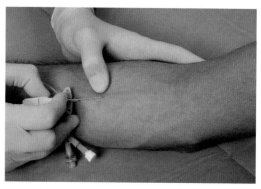

Fig. 8.2 Insert needle at a 20–30 degrees angle to the skin, with the bevel facing upwards.

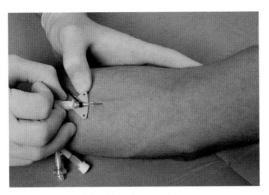

Fig. 8.3   Look for a flashback of blood into the cannula.

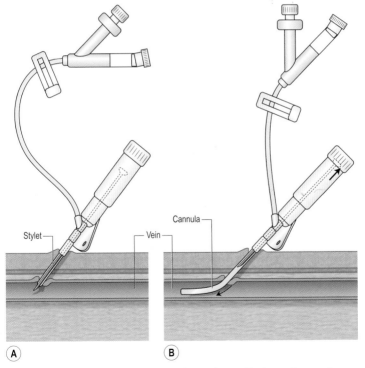

Stylet

Cannula

Vein

(A)

(B)

Fig. 8.4   (A) Once the tip of the cannula is in the vein lumen, (B) advance the cannula over the stylet which is held stationary.

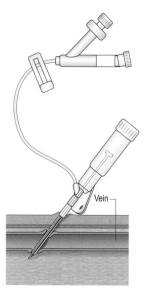

Fig. 8.5 If no blood flows into the cannula after the initial flashback it may have transfixed the vein (passed through the opposite side).

 Tip Box

If flashback is initially seen but upon withdrawing the stylet slightly blood does not flow into the cannula, the vein may have been transfixed by your initial puncture (Fig. 8.5).

To try to save the situation, pull the cannula back very slowly whilst watching for flashback. When it returns into the vein lumen now try to advance gently, sliding the cannula into the vein. This is often best done with a 2 mL syringe filled with saline attached to the cannula and delicately flushing some saline as the cannula is slowly advanced. If a bleb appears it is better to stop and start afresh.

- Release tourniquet.
- Remove the needle and attach a three-way tap pre-filled with normal saline.
- Clean away any residual blood from the area and place a clear dressing over the cannula site.
- Flush the cannula with 10 mL normal saline.

Tip Box
Ensure the clear part of the cannula plaster is over the puncture site to ensure irritation and areas of cellulitis or erythema are noted early.

Tip Box
- If there is any discomfort when the normal saline flush is administered or the cannula does not flush easily, remove the cannula.
- Once under the skin and the stylet has been partially withdrawn from within the plastic cannula, never re-sheath the cannula with the stylet. This risks shearing off the end of the cannula with the stylet under the skin.
- Resistance encountered when sliding the cannula into the vein despite observing flashback may be due to a valve within the vein – more often than not this situation is irretrievable. Try applying traction to the skin with your non-dominant hand whilst sliding in the cannula, but take care that this does not cause discomfort to the patient.
- If you fail the patient will not be very disposed to further multiple attempts. Either ask someone more experienced or prior to subsequent attempts apply local anaesthetics particularly if a large cannula is needed.

POST-PROCEDURE CARE

- Date the cannula on the plaster (most hospitals have a policy of removing a cannula after 48 hours to prevent cannula-related cellulitis).
- Ask the nursing staff to bandage the cannula if the patient is confused and prone to pulling at their lines (but ensure that the site is regularly checked for local infection).

COMPLICATIONS

- Failed cannulation.
- Cannula cellulitis or thrombophlebitis (remove cannula and consider empirical antibiotics and analgesia).
- Air embolism – ensure that the cannula fills with blood prior to attaching the sterile bung or three-way tap.

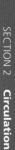

SECTION 2 **Circulation**

CHAPTER 9

PREPARING AND SETTING UP INTRAVENOUS MEDICATIONS

INTRODUCTION

Intravenous fluids or medication for administration are usually prepared by nursing staff. However, junior doctors should be able to perform this simple task.

INDICATIONS

- Administration of intravenous fluids.
- Administration of intravenous medications.
- Intravenous replacement of electrolytes.

CONTRAINDICATIONS

- Cellulitis at the cannula site – replace the cannula elsewhere if suspected (see Chapter 8).

EQUIPMENT

- Intravenous bag of fluid, e.g. normal saline, 5% dextrose.
- Intravenous giving set and drip stand.
- Gauze.
- Gloves.

PRACTICAL PROCEDURE

- Wash your hands and wear gloves.
- Open the intravenous giving set from its sterile packaging.
- Place the intravenous bag of fluid on fluid stand.
- Check the cannula site to ensure it is free from local infection and the use-by date on the bag of fluid.
- Twist off the plastic end of the access port on the fluid bag.
- Carefully push the sharp plastic bevel of the giving set into the access port of the bag of fluid, taking care not to touch the bevel and thus maintain sterility (Fig. 9.1). Allow fluid to run into the giving set chamber by opening the roller clamp (Fig. 9.2).
- Fluid should be allowed to run from the giving set chamber through the administration set tubing until air bubbles are flushed out. The roller clamp can then be closed to halt further flow.
- Remove the bung from the already sited intravenous cannula and flush the cannula with 10 mL of sterile normal saline to ensure patency and intravenous placement.
- Attach the end of the giving set to the cannula and open the giving set up again.
- Observe the giving set chamber. A steady flow of drips confirms free flow of fluid through the giving set, which can be adjusted by manipulating the roller mechanism on the giving set.

Tip Box

Calculate the rate of the infusion in drops per minute (dpm) using the following formula:

$$\frac{\text{Fluid volume (ml)}}{\text{Infusion time (hours)}} \quad X \quad \frac{20 \text{ (number of drops per ml in a standard giving set)}}{60 \text{ (rate per minute)}}$$

For example, for a 1 L bag of intravenous fluids over 8 hours:

$$\frac{1000}{8} \quad X \quad \frac{20}{60} \quad = \quad 42 \text{ dpm}$$

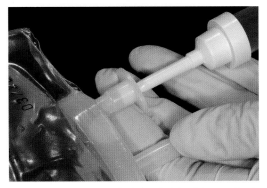

Fig. 9.1   Do not touch the sharp, sterile plastic bevel of the giving set when inserting into the fluid bag.

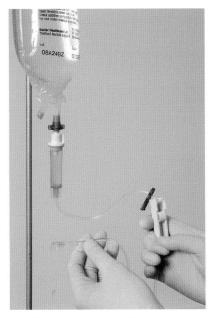

Fig. 9.2   Open the roller clamp, allowing fluid into the giving set.

- Ensure that the bag of fluid is kept hanging above the patient to avoid retrograde flow of blood into the giving set.
- If the fluid fails to run through, check the giving set for kinks. If this fails to work, disconnect the giving set from the cannula and manipulate the position of the intravenous cannula. Try flushing the cannula with saline to confirm patency and intravenous position, then reconnect to the giving set.

COMPLICATIONS

- Air embolism. Air bubbles in the plastic giving set tubing may be inadvertently flushed intravenously. Patients with patent intracardiac foramina may be at risk of paradoxical arterial embolic events. This problem can be avoided by opening the giving set to allow free flow of fluid until all bubbles are flushed out. Alternatively tap the giving set tubing until air bubbles rise through the tubing and dissipate within the giving set chamber.
- Poor fluid flow associated with new pain at the cannula insertion site usually means subcutaneous extravasated fluid with the cannula no longer in situ. Consider replacing the cannula if in situ repositioning does not resolve the problem.

CHAPTER 10

INTRAVENOUS FLUIDS AND COMMONLY PRESCRIBED INFUSIONS

Dr Thomas Aitchison Latta (circa 1790–1833) pioneered the use of intravenous saline as fluid resuscitation for cholera victims in 1832 using a small silver tube attached to a syringe.

INTRODUCTION

Fluid balance and the prescription of intravenous fluids is one of the most common duties performed by a hospital doctor. A detailed explanation of the physiology underlying fluid balance is beyond the scope of this text, but it is imperative that fluid prescriptions are based upon the individual requirements of that patient; there is no such thing as a standard fluid regimen. The patient should have their fluid status assessed through clinical history and examination prior to determining their management (Table 10.1).

A strictly documented fluid balance chart, if accurate, might be helpful in assessing the prescription of intravenous fluids. However, third-space sequestration, gastrointestinal losses and febrile illnesses, for example, may lead to a gross underestimate of losses and what may appear to be a positive balance on paper due to modest fluid administration can in fact be very misleading. Remember a patient's clinical signs never lie, and should be relied upon in preference to a fluid balance.

Furthermore, the clinical assessment should be made in the context of the patient's acute disorder and chronic co-morbidities:

- Some common causes of hypovolaemia include:
  - insensible losses, e.g. febrile illness and lack of fluid intake
  - third space losses, e.g. bowel obstruction, sepsis, ascites
  - acute losses, e.g. profuse diarrhoea (especially secondary to *Clostridium difficile*), vomiting, haemorrhage
  - excessive diuresis, whether drug-induced or secondary to diabetes mellitus or insipidus.

SECTION 2 **Circulation**

TABLE 10.1 Indicators of fluid status from the history and examination

	Hypovolaemia	Fluid overload
Symptoms	Thirst Headache Dark, concentrated urine Oliguria	Dyspnoea Orthopnoea Frothy (white/pink) sputum
Signs in order of frequency and reliability	Tachycardia Hypotension Cool peripheries Prolonged capillary refill time (>2 seconds) Postural hypotension (systolic drop of >20 mmHg on rising) Low jugular venous pressure Dry mucous membranes Increased skin turgor Sunken eyes	Tachypnoea Tachycardia Relative hypertension Low oxygen saturations Raised JVP Bilateral crepitations (initially bibasal but rising depending upon the degree of pulmonary oedema) Third heart sound (gallop rhythm) Peripheral oedema (dependent areas such as ankles and sacrum. Not reliable in the presence of concomitant hypoalbuminaemia)
Investigations	High urine specific gravity (concentrated urine) Oliguria/anuria Raised urea (initially) and creatinine (later) Raised serum osmolality Rising base deficit	Chest X-ray features of pulmonary oedema

- Chronic co-morbidities requiring judicious fluid input:
  — left ventricular failure
  — end-stage renal failure
  — ascites.

DEHYDRATION VERSUS HYPOVOLAEMIA

While dehydration is commonly a term used to mean hypovolaemia the two are different. Dehydration is a relative loss of water that will lead to hypernatraemia and hyperuricaemia, while hypovolaemia is loss of circulating volume regardless of the fluid loss (blood, sequestration due to sepsis, GI fluid losses, etc.) and may or may not be associated with sodium and urea changes. The mechanism for urea change in hypovolaemic patients is as much related to renal hypoperfusion as it is to the composition of the fluid loss. Only the respiratory system leads to a pure water loss while diarrhoea leads to a relatively increased water loss.

Furthermore, it is possible for a patient to be normovolaemic and dehydrated or hypovolaemic and dehydrated. The former is often seen in hospitalized patients whose insensible losses are only replaced with saline. Consequently it is important for management purposes to be clear when describing dehydration, hypovolaemia or both.

INTRAVENOUS FLUIDS

Intravenous fluids can be divided into two types, namely crystalloids and colloids.

Crystalloids

Crystalloid solutions are aqueous solutions containing electrolytes that pass freely across semipermeable membranes. Crystalloids have no oncotic pressure, and so distribute readily from the intravascular compartment to the interstitium and beyond. For this reason crystalloids such as normal saline are commonly used for maintenance intravenous fluid replacement. The type of maintenance fluids prescribed needs to be tailored to the individual requirements of the patient taking into account both their volume status and electrolyte requirements (Table 10.2).

- 5% dextrose is an isotonic solution that can effectively be thought of as intravenous water, because once infused the dextrose is metabolized. The dextrose serves to maintain tonicity and therefore prevents immediate red blood cell haemolysis. In effect the solution provides pure water and therefore will reduce urea and sodium concentrations. It is distributed throughout the whole body water (intracellular and extracellular). Consequently it is the least efficient fluid for intravascular volume replenishment.
- Hartmann's solution contains less chloride than normal saline, 5 mmol/L of potassium and 29 mmol/L of lactate, which is later converted in the liver to bicarbonate. Thus Hartmann's solution is more representative of plasma and so is described as being more 'physiological'. This solution is distributed to the extracellular space (i.e. the interstitial and intravascular compartments).
- Normal saline is also exclusively distributed to the extracellular space and is as effective as Hartmann's solution for restoring intravascular volume. If used exclusively it will lead to a rise in serum sodium and because of the chloride content produce hyperchloraemia, which displaces bicarbonate and thus may be responsible for a mild metabolic acidosis.

TABLE 10.2 Crystalloid solutions vary in their electrolyte concentrations (mmol/L)

	Na^+	K^+	Cl^-	Ca^{2+}	lactate
Normal saline (NaCl 0.9%)	154	–	154	–	–
NaCl 0.45%	77	–	77	–	–
Dextrose–saline (NaCl 0.18%, dextrose 4%)	30	–	30	–	–
Dextrose 5%	–	–	–	–	–
Hartmann's solution	131	5	111	2	29
Ringer's solution	130	4	109	1.5	28

Colloids

In comparison to crystalloids, colloids are large molecules that contribute to oncotic pressure and do not cross semi-permeable membranes. In reality colloids simply remain within the intravascular compartment for longer than crystalloids, hence the use of solutions containing colloid for the rapid and acute expansion of intravascular volume (e.g. haemorrhage). In situations of increased capillary permeability, such as sepsis, colloids will eventually leak across the capillary membrane causing interstitial oedema through raising the interstitial oncotic pressure.

- Colloid solutions contain either natural colloid (e.g. blood products) or synthetic colloid.
- Gelatin-containing solutions include Haemaccel and Gelofusine, whereas Dextran contains high-molecular-weight dextrose.
- Colloids have the disadvantages of being considerably more expensive than crystalloids and can on rare occasions cause anaphylactic reactions (more so with Dextran).
- Blood is the only colloid with oxygen-carrying capacity.

CRYSTALLOID VERSUS COLLOID: WHICH FLUID TO USE IN THE CRITICALLY ILL?

Inadequate tissue perfusion in the critically ill patient leads to anaerobic metabolism within those tissues, commonly manifesting as peripherally cool and shutdown extremities with a progressively worsening base deficit. Therefore rapid volume resuscitation is required to restore adequate tissue perfusion.

Medical opinion still varies regarding the fluid of choice in these circumstances. However, the essence of managing hypovolaemia is rapid restoration of circulating volume and although the various solutions may have differing theoretical efficiencies, in practice it is ensuring the initiation of the process that matters as much as the type of fluid used. Giving orders to start administering a colloid that does not take place for an hour is significantly worse than starting immediate resuscitation with 5% dextrose!

The choice of fluid is in part influenced by what is at hand, the speed of fluid loss and the type of fluid loss. For example:

- profuse diarrhoea can be managed with moderately rapid infusions of dextrose saline and 5% dextrose
- rapid blood loss, which has a more immediate effect on circulating volume, might be better managed with very rapid colloid (likely to be more effective) and crystalloid solutions, or blood if immediately available. The importance in this situation is the speed of infusion.

FLUID CHALLENGES

If the aim of fluid administration is to determine whether hypovolaemia is the cause of new clinical signs such as oliguria, a colloid fluid challenge of between 300 and 500 mL over 30 minutes would be more effective in restoring normality than a similar quantity of saline. Colloid fluid challenges are therefore more likely to reveal whether hypovolaemia was indeed the reason for the change in clinical signs.

DAILY FLUID REQUIREMENTS

In health an average 70-kg adult requires 3 L of fluid per day for the maintenance of euvolaemia, with approximately 40–60 mmol of potassium and 100 mmol of sodium. It is worth noting that a proportion of these fluid and electrolyte requirements come from foods as well as fluids. For example, an otherwise fit and well 70-kg individual who is nil by mouth prior to an elective surgical procedure would reasonably have a 24-hour maintenance fluid regimen as in Table 10.3.

As described above, the volume and constitution of a patient's fluid requirements in illness will vary depending upon both their volume status and the nature of the underlying disease process.

TABLE 10.3 Fluid regimen for an average (70-kg) adult who is nil by mouth

Date	Fluid	Quantity	Additives	Quantity	Rate	Route
28/6	5% dextrose	1 L			8 hours	i.v.
28/6	0.9% saline	1 L	KCl	40 mmol	8 hours	i.v.
28/6	5% dextrose	1 L			8 hours	i.v.

ELECTROLYTE REQUIREMENTS: SPECIAL CIRCUMSTANCES

A detailed explanation of electrolyte physiology is again beyond the scope of this text, but it is important to appreciate certain pathological states in which important caveats exist to the prescription of electrolytes.

Heart and liver failure

These are states that exhibit pathological over-activity of the renin–angiotensin cascade. Thus sodium intake should be restricted in these groups of patients in addition to close monitoring of their overall fluid balance. Many centres advise 5% dextrose as a maintenance fluid of choice in hepatic failure.

SECTION 2 Circulation

Chronic renal failure

Patients with chronic renal failure will have an impaired ability to both produce urine and excrete potassium in their urine. Therefore potassium supplementation should be avoided in these patients (especially with end-stage renal failure) unless levels are dangerously low.

Diabetic ketoacidosis

This characteristically presents with metabolic acidosis, hyperglycaemia, hypovolaemia and dehydration due to a urinary sugar osmotic diuresis, and hyperkalaemia due to a lack of insulin. It is typically managed initially with rapid saline resuscitation and an intravenous insulin sliding scale until blood sugars come close to the normal range. Although such patients may have high initial serum potassium concentrations, overall total body potassium levels are depleted due to the osmotic diuresis. The subsequent administration of insulin and correction of metabolic acidosis will return potassium to its intracellular sites and serum potassium will fall. In this acute circumstance, a potassium infusion via a central venous line with close monitoring of potassium levels will be necessary once an insulin sliding scale has been started to avoid precipitously falling potassium levels.

Large gastrointestinal losses

Patients in whom hypovolaemia and associated dehydration occurs secondary to large gastrointestinal losses will also require intravenous replacement of lost potassium and magnesium.

Large urinary losses

Patients receiving diuretics will concomitantly excrete sodium, potassium and magnesium in their urine to varying degrees. If blood levels start falling, potassium and magnesium both require replacement to avoid complications (especially arrhythmias).

- If diuretics are being administered to treat fluid overload, potassium should be supplemented orally.
- Avoid oral magnesium preparations as these are particularly prone to causing diarrhoea as a side-effect. Even in fluid overload, magnesium is more effectively replaced intravenously in very small volumes of fluid (as little as 20 mL – see Intravenous fluids section).
- In contrast, hyponatraemia secondary to diuretic use is resolved simply by cutting back on the diuretic medications rather than replacing sodium.

Arrhythmias

The prevention and treatment of arrhythmias involves ensuring that potassium and magnesium levels are adequately controlled. Both are predominantly intracellular ions closely involved in cardiac rhythm generation and conduction. Low extracellular levels (detected on blood analysis) should be corrected in the management of arrhythmias. Aim for a serum potassium of >4.5 mmol/L, with serum magnesium >1.0 mmol/L. Take care to avoid fluid overload whilst replacing these electrolytes in the presence of a tachyarrhythmia.

Refeeding syndrome

This can occur in previously starved/malnourished patients in whom enteral feeding has been resumed. Carbohydrate administration stimulates insulin release, with the depletion of extracellular potassium, magnesium and phosphate levels following their shift into the intracellular environment. Avoidance of this condition can be achieved with daily monitoring and replacement of potassium, magnesium and phosphate whilst feeding is introduced under the guidance of a dietitian.

COMMONLY PRESCRIBED INFUSIONS

INSULIN SLIDING SCALE

This is indicated in several situations:

- the treatment of diabetic ketoacidosis (DKA) or hyperosmolar non-ketosis (HONK)
- in diabetic patients who are nil by mouth pre-operatively or pre-procedure (e.g. oesophagogastroduodenoscopy (OGD))
- intercurrent illness requiring tight blood sugar control (e.g. sepsis, acute coronary syndromes).

The sliding scale in Table 10.4 is one example of how to prescribe the insulin regimen, but check to see if your hospital already has a local policy in place.

GLYCERYL TRINITRATE (GTN) INFUSION

See Table 10.5 for an example of a GTN infusion prescription.

Indications include:

- ongoing cardiac chest pain despite initial management (e.g. GTN spray)
- the management of acute pulmonary oedema.

AMIODARONE INFUSION

See Table 10.6 for an example of an amiodarone infusion prescription. Indications include:

- supraventricular, nodal and ventricular tachycardias
- atrial fibrillation and flutter (for chemical cardioversion in the presence of structural heart disease)
- ventricular fibrillation (in this case amiodarone would be given as a stat 300 mg dose as part of the cardiac arrest protocol).

TABLE 10.4 An example of an insulin sliding scale regimen

Date	Fluid	Quantity	Additives	Quantity	Rate	Route
28/6	0.9% saline	50 mL	Actrapid	50 units	See chart	i.v.
	CBGM	**Rate (units/hour)**				
	0–4.0	Stop				
	4.1–8.0	1				
	8.1–12.0	2				
	12.1–14.0	3				
	14.1–16.0	4				
	16.1–20.0	5				
	>20	Call Dr				
28/6	0.9% saline	1 L	If BM >15		8 hours	i.v.
28/6	5% dextrose	1 L	If BM <15		8 hours	i.v.

Adjust the insulin infusion rate according to blood sugar measurement.
Note that in the case of DKA, the fluid regimen will be different to that attached to the above standard sliding scale regimen.
CBGM, capillary blood glucose monitoring; DKA, diabetic ketoacidosis.

TABLE 10.5 An example of a prescription for glyceryl trinitrate (GTN)

Date	Fluid	Quantity	Additives	Quantity	Rate	Route
28/6	0.9% saline	50 mL	GTN*	50 mg	See below	i.v.

Titrate infusion rate to symptoms and systolic BP. Aim for systolic BP >110

*GTN is a potent vasodilator. The infusion must thus be started at a low rate and be titrated against the systolic BP, which can fall precipitously with GTN. Therefore start the infusion at 1–2 mL/hour, re-check the BP and increase the infusion rate accordingly.

TABLE 10.6 An example of a prescription for amiodarone

Date	Fluid	Quantity	Additives	Quantity	Rate	Route
28/6	5% glucose	100 mL	Amiodarone	300 mg	1 hour	i.v.
28/6	5% glucose	1 L	Amiodarone	900 mg	23 hours	i.v.
29/6	5% glucose	1 L	Amiodarone	900 mg	24 hours	i.v.

The following points should be noted with intravenous amiodarone:

- Optimize electrolytes prior to starting anti-arrhythmic therapy.
- Telemetry is required with amiodarone infusions to monitor clinical response.
- The 1-hour intravenous loading dose of amiodarone can initially (in emergency situations) be given peripherally via a large-bore cannula, but should be continued via a central venous line.
- Check baseline liver function tests and thyroid function tests prior to starting amiodarone, as deranged liver and thyroid function may ensue.
- After the first 24 hours, subsequent 900 mg/24 hour infusions are only given if necessary according to clinical response. If clinical response has been achieved, switch to p.o. amiodarone.

PHENYTOIN INFUSION

Indications include (check with senior prior to starting):

- status epilepticus (i.e. refractory to initial benzodiazepine therapy)
- seizures (or seizure prophylaxis) in neurosurgery.

The loading dose of intravenous phenytoin is *15 mg/kg at a rate not exceeding 50 mg/min*. Therefore Table 10.7 is a prescription for a phenytoin infusion for a 70-kg man.

- Telemetry is required with phenytoin infusions to monitor for arrhythmias.
- Monitor phenytoin infusions by measurement of plasma phenytoin levels.

TABLE 10.7 An example of a prescription for a phenytoin infusion for a 70-kg man

Date	Fluid	Quantity	Additives	Quantity	Rate	Route
28/6	0.9% saline	100 mL	Phenytoin	1050 mg	25 minutes (4 mL/minute)	i.v.
28/6	0.9% saline	100 mL	Phenytoin	100 mg	6–8 hours	i.v.

AMINOPHYLLINE INFUSION

Indications include (check with senior prior to starting):

- reversible airways obstruction (e.g. chronic obstructive pulmonary disease with demonstrated reversibility)
- acute severe asthma.

Note

- Patients taking oral aminophylline or theophylline should not receive intravenous aminophylline unless plasma theophylline concentration is available to guide dosage.
- In patients not previously taking aminophylline or theophylline, a loading dose is given at 5 mg/kg (between 250 and 500 mg) over at least 20 minutes. A subsequent maintenance infusion is given at 500 μg/kg/hour, adjusted according to plasma theophylline concentration.

Table 10.8 is a prescription for an aminophylline infusion for a 70-kg man not previously taking aminophylline or theophylline.

- Telemetry is required with aminophylline infusions to monitor for arrhythmias.
- Monitor aminophylline infusions by measurement of plasma aminophylline levels.

TABLE 10.8 An example of a prescription for an aminophylline infusion for a 70-kg man (previously aminophylline naive)

Date	Fluid	Quantity	Additives	Quantity	Rate	Route
28/6	0.9% saline	100 mL	Aminophylline	350 mg	30 minutes	i.v.
28/6	0.9% saline	500 mL	Aminophylline	280 mg	8 hours	i.v.

MAGNESIUM INFUSION

Indications include (check with senior prior to starting – see Table 10.9):

- hypomagnesaemia (commonly encountered in sepsis, diuretic use, diarrhoea, chronic alcohol excess, refeeding syndrome), a common precipitant of cardiac arrhythmias
- acute severe asthma not responding to initial nebulized bronchodilators.

TABLE 10.9 An example of a prescription for intravenous magnesium

Date	Fluid	Quantity	Additives	Quantity	Rate	Route
28/6	0.9% saline	100 mL	Magnesium	2 g (8 mmol)	20 minutes	i.v.

CENTRAL VENOUS CATHETER INSERTION

Stephen Hales (1677–1761) performed the first recorded central venous catheterization in 1733 when he inserted a glass tube into the jugular vein of a horse to measure central venous pressure. In 1953 Seldinger described a percutaneous method for central venous access, and subsequently central venous cannulation became a widespread medical technique.

INTRODUCTION

Modern central venous catheters have several lumen, which allow for:

- infusion of drugs (such as concentrated potassium solutions and inotropes)
- convenient repeated central venous blood sampling for investigations such as blood gas analysis
- measurement of central venous pressure (CVP), which contributes to the assessment of intravascular volume status.

SECTION 2   Circulation

Central venous catheters can be placed in the internal jugular, subclavian or femoral veins using the Seldinger technique. This chapter will discuss internal jugular and femoral approaches.

NICE GUIDELINES ON ULTRASOUND GUIDANCE

- 2D imaging ultrasound guidance should be the preferred method when inserting a central venous catheter in adults and children in elective situations.
- 2D imaging ultrasound guidance should be considered in most clinical situations, either elective or emergency, where central venous catheter insertion is necessary.
- When using the ultrasound, ensure that the orientation of the probe correlates with the anatomical position. The probe head should have a marker on one side that corresponds to a marker on the screen, enabling the user to identify correct orientation of the probe (and hence correct orientation of the vessels you are visualizing!).
- Having found the internal jugular or femoral vessels, check for the vein by compressing the region with the probe. The vein collapses with the application of pressure whereas the thicker-walled artery remains patent and pulsates (Fig. 11.1A and B).

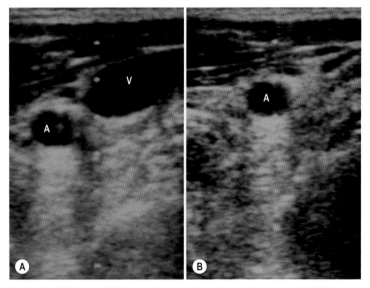

Fig. 11.1   (A) Ultrasound of the carotid artery (*A*) and internal jugular vein (*V*). (B) The internal jugular vein collapses with gentle compression of the ultrasound probe against the neck, leaving the pulsatile carotid artery (*A*).

INDICATIONS

- Measurement of central venous pressure.
- Secure intravenous access in patients requiring several lumens for i.v. infusions.
- Pre-operatively for major operations, e.g. aortic aneurysm repair, coronary artery bypass grafts; these are usually inserted by anaesthetists.

CONTRAINDICATIONS

- Coagulopathy (relative contraindication).
- Local sepsis over puncture site.
- Lack of consent.

EQUIPMENT

- Dressing pack.
- Sterile gown, gloves and drapes.
- Chlorhexidine cleaning solution.
- Lidocaine.
- 2 × 10 mL syringes.
- 1 × 5 mL syringe.
- Orange needle.
- 2 × green needles.
- Sterile gauze.
- 100 mL sterile bag normal saline.
- Central line pack (includes central line, introducer needle, guidewire and dilator).
- 3-way taps (the quantity corresponding to the number of lumens on the central line).
- Scalpel.
- Suture.
- Clear sterile dressing.
- If available – portable ultrasound probe, sterile cover and probe jelly.

PRACTICAL PROCEDURE

- Obtain consent.
- Ask a nurse to accompany you in order to open non-sterile equipment and to comfort the patient.

POSITIONING FOR INTERNAL JUGULAR LINE PLACEMENT

- Lay the patient flat on the bed and elevate the bed to your level for your own comfort.
- Tilt the bed with the head down (the Trendelenburg position). This reduces the risk of air embolism whilst also helping to distend the neck veins.

Tip Box

If the patient is more dyspnoeic in the head-down position, minimize the time spent in this position by performing the skin preparation and infiltration of local anaesthesia with the patient sitting up.

- Turn the patient's head approximately 30 degrees from the midline away from the side of line insertion.

Tip Box

If the patient is inadvertently flexing their neck, place a 0.5- or 1-L bag of normal saline between the shoulder blades; this allows for more neck extension.

Tip Box

Place the patient on telemetry in order to observe for potential arrhythmias during insertion. These occur if the guidewire or line is inserted too far and makes contact with the tricuspid valve, in which case pull back the guidewire.

PREPARATION

- Wash hands, wear the sterile gown and gloves and lay out sterile environment and dressing pack.
- Check and assemble the equipment – attach three-way taps to all lumens of the central line other than the port through which the guidewire will pass. Flush the ports with normal saline to ensure patency (simply pierce the sterile bag of normal saline with a green needle attached to a 10 mL syringe and withdraw saline as required). Once flushed, turn the 3-way taps off to the patient.

Tip Box

After flushing the lines, keep the saline flush syringe on top of the normal saline so as not to confuse it with the lidocaine syringe.

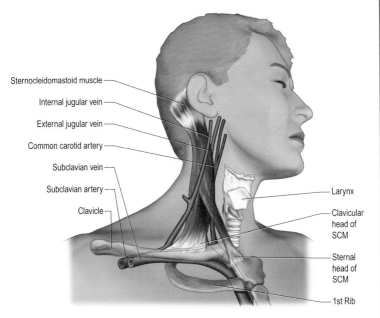

Fig. 11.2 Landmarks at the anterior triangle of the neck for central venous catheter insertion. SCM, sternocleidomastoid.

Labels (top to bottom, left): Sternocleidomastoid muscle; Internal jugular vein; External jugular vein; Common carotid artery; Subclavian vein; Subclavian artery; Clavicle. (right): Larynx; Clavicular head of SCM; Sternal head of SCM; 1st Rib

- Clean the area – clean outwards in a spiral motion from the centre to the periphery.
- Place a sterile drape over the patient with a central window over the area of line insertion.
- Palpate the carotid artery and ultrasound the area in order to obtain a guide of the anatomy and landmarks for insertion (Fig. 11.2).
- The surface point at which the line enters the neck is midway between the sternal notch and the mastoid process, lateral to the carotid pulsation. The line subsequently advances under the sternocleidomastoid muscle towards the internal jugular vein.

STERILE TECHNIQUE FOR SETTING UP THE ULTRASOUND PROBE

- The operator rolls up the sterile plastic sheath into a 'sock' whilst an assistant applies gel onto the ultrasound probe head.
- Offer the sterile sheath to the assistant who can then place the probe into the sheath (Fig. 11.3). In this way the sterile operator does not touch the non-sterile probe, and likewise the non-sterile assistant does not contaminate the sterile sheath.
- Roll the sheath down to its full length and secure with the sterile elastic bands around the probe head (Fig. 11.4). The probe is now sterile and can be placed on the sterile trolley or on your sterile field.

SECTION 2 **Circulation**

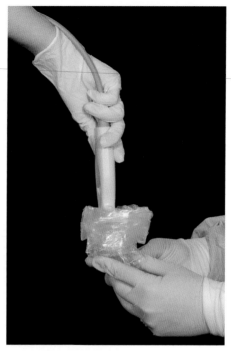

Fig. 11.3 Offer the sterile sheath to the assistant who can then place the probe head into the sheath.

- Chlorhexidine cleaning solution applied to the sterile probe head is an excellent transducer, and avoids the need for gel in your sterile field. Once the sterile plastic sheath is secured, simply dip the sterile probe head into a gallipot of alcoholic chlorhexidine solution and subsequently apply the sterile probe head to the patient's skin to obtain an image.
- When using the ultrasound, identify the internal jugular vein and align the probe with the vein in the centre of your picture. When inserting the needle below the probe head aim directly for the internal jugular vein on the screen.

PROCEDURE

- Infiltrate local anaesthetic subcutaneously with the orange needle. Ensure you pull back before injecting anaesthetic ensuring no venous delivery.
- Infiltrate local anaesthetic with the green needle into deeper tissues.

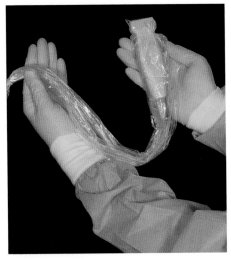

Fig. 11.4   Roll the sheath down to its full length and secure with the sterile elastic bands around the probe head.

Tip Box

Some operators advocate the use of a 'guide needle'. The internal jugular vein is deliberately located when infiltrating local anaesthetic. Upon puncture of the vein, the syringe is removed from the needle, which is left in situ as a marker of the vein's location.

Tip Box

Loosen the guidewire ensuring it runs smoothly in and out of its sheath and place it next to you on the sterile drape so that it is readily accessible. The shorter the time between venepuncture and introducing the guidewire, the greater the chance of success.

- Connect the 5 mL syringe to the introducer needle.
- At the same time as palpating the carotid pulse (or preferably whilst using ultrasound guidance), insert the syringe at the point midway between the sternal notch and the mastoid process, lateral to the carotid pulsation (Fig. 11.5). Aim towards the ipsilateral nipple advancing under the sternocleidomastoid whilst continuously aspirating for blood.

SECTION 2 **Circulation**

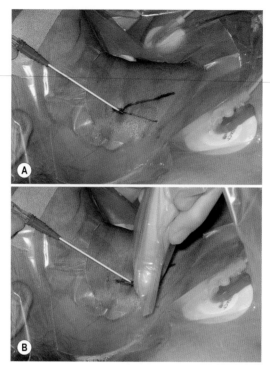

Fig. 11.5 (A, B) At the same time as palpating the carotid pulse or preferably while using ultrasound guidance, insert the syringe at the point midway between the sternal notch and the mastoid process, lateral to the carotid pulsation.

Tip Box

Distinguishing features between venous and arterial puncture may include (for arterial puncture) pulsatile flow and a brighter colour of blood. However, these features are not to be relied upon, and if you are in any doubt as to the nature of the vessel punctured remove the needle immediately and apply firm compression. Re-try preferably under ultrasound guidance.

- Having located and confirmed the vein by blood aspiration into the syringe (Fig. 11.6) hold the needle still with the non-dominant hand and remove the syringe with the other.

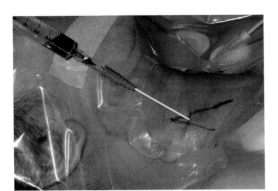

Fig. 11.6   Aspirating blood upon internal jugular venous puncture.

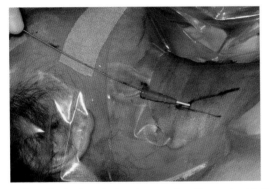

Fig. 11.7   Pass the guidewire down the introducer needle until approximately 10 cm of wire have passed into the vein.

- Pass the guidewire down the introducer needle with the dominant hand ensuring that some 10 cm of wire have passed into the vein (Fig. 11.7). Keep a close eye on the telemetry and watch for arrhythmias. Should these occur pull the guidewire back until the arrhythmia terminates.

Tip Box

NEVER force the guidewire through the needle if significant resistance is felt. Remove the guidewire and recheck that the tip of the introducer needle still lies in the lumen of the vein.

SECTION 2   **Circulation**

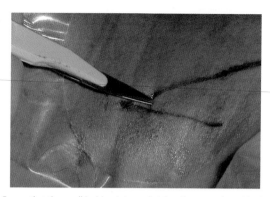

Fig. 11.8   Ensure that the small incision is immediately adjacent to the guidewire to avoid a 'skin bridge' between the guidewire and the incision.

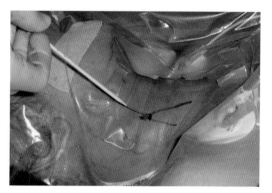

Fig. 11.9   Pass the dilator over the guidewire.

- Ensuring that you do not lose sight of the guidewire at any time, remove the needle over the guidewire.
- While moving the tail of the guidewire to one side, make a small (approximately 0.5 cm) incision with the scalpel in the skin to enlarge the guidewire's percutaneous passage. Ensure that the incision is immediately adjacent to the guidewire to avoid a 'skin bridge' between the guidewire and the incision (Fig. 11.8).
- Pass the dilator over the guidewire (Fig. 11.9), and advance under the skin once the guidewire has reappeared at the other end of the dilator.
- Whilst holding the guidewire at its tip, advance the dilator through the skin (the small incision accommodating the girth of the dilator). This usually needs a firm advance with a slight rotating motion to pass through skin into the vein.

Tip Box

The ease of passage of the dilator not only depends upon skin elasticity and the size of the nick in the skin, but sometimes if difficult it might indicate inadvertent passage through the internal carotid arterial wall. Be suspicious of this complication if it is difficult to pass the dilator, especially if the guidewire seems to be well in situ and moves freely without kinks. If any concern exists regarding arterial placement of the guidewire and/or dilator, remove the apparatus and apply firm pressure with gauze over the area for 5 to 10 minutes.

- Once a path has been dilated remove the dilator over the guidewire, taking care to not remove the guidewire at the same time. Now cover the enlarged puncture site with gauze to guard against air embolism.
- Pass the central line over the guidewire, ensuring that the guidewire appears from the other end before the central line touches the skin (Fig. 11.10). In most multi-lumen catheters the guidewire appears through the brown capped channel.
- Whilst holding the guidewire at its tip, advance the central line through the skin along the dilated passage. There should be no sense of resistance.
- Insert the line to 15 cm.
- Place the suture cover on the line at the point of entry to the skin (15 cm).
- Suture the line in place both at the suture cover and at the neck of the line to reduce movement of the venous catheter (Fig. 11.11).
- Check all lumens aspirate and flush freely. Turn the 3-way tap 'off' to the patient.
- Apply a clear sterile dressing over the line (Fig. 11.12).
- Document the procedure clearly in the patient's medical notes.

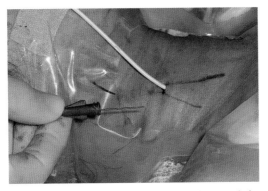

Fig. 11.10   Ensure that the guidewire appears from the central line port before advancing the central line.

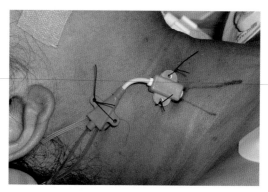

Fig. 11.11 Suture the line at the suture cover and at the neck of the line.

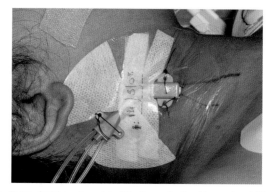

Fig. 11.12 Ensure that the entry-point of the line under the skin remains visible.

PLACEMENT OF FEMORAL LINES

This differs from the internal jugular in a number of ways.

- The patient does not need to be lying head down or need to be monitored.
- Location (see Fig. 6.5) is easier by palpation of the femoral artery (located at the midpoint between the anterior superior iliac spine and the pubic symphysis) with the vein located medially (whereas the internal jugular vein is lateral to the artery in the neck). Use of ultrasound simplifies vein location.
- Once the femoral vein is located the venous catheter can be inserted to its full length using the same technique described above and sutured in place.
- Given the proximity to areas with numerous microbes, the preparation and maintenance of sterility is extremely important. Femoral lines are more likely to become infected and therefore tend to have a shorter life span.

COMPLICATIONS

- Infection.
- Bleeding and haematoma formation (in neck or retroperitoneum depending upon site of insertion).
- Pneumothorax (internal jugular).
- Arterial puncture: should this occur, remove the needle and apply firm compression for at least 5 minutes.
- Venous thrombosis.

POST-PROCEDURE INVESTIGATIONS AND CARE

- For internal jugular lines use a chest X-ray to check line position and rule out pneumothorax. Internal jugular lines should be sited with the tip at the junction of the superior vena cava/right atrium.
- Central venous blood gas analysis central venous oxygen saturations are commonly used in the critical care environment.
- Sepsis in the presence of an indwelling central venous catheter warrants insertion of a line elsewhere and removal of the current line. Send blood cultures both from the central line and peripherally. Send the tip of the venous catheter in a sterile container to microbiology upon removal.
- Central venous pressure monitoring if in the internal jugular position. This may be performed using either:
  — a direct electronic transducer system with the central venous pressure (CVP) reading and waveform displayed on a monitor or
  — a manometer containing crystalloid attached to the internal jugular line.

MEASURING CENTRAL VENOUS PRESSURE USING A MANOMETER

Once the internal jugular catheter is in situ, arranging the apparatus to measure CVP would be a task expected of the nursing staff on the ward. As this procedure is performed infrequently in the ward setting, however, this may not always be the case. It is therefore important to have some knowledge about how to set up the manometer to obtain accurate CVP readings.

EQUIPMENT

- Sterile gloves.
- 1 L bag of normal saline.
- Giving set.
- 3-way tap.

- Extension tubing.
- CVP manometer.
- Drip stand.
- Skin pen.
- Spirit level.

PRACTICAL PROCEDURE

- Wash your hands and wear sterile gloves.
- Ensure that the central venous catheter aspirates and flushes freely. Use the distal port for CVP measurement.
- Connect a 3-way tap to:
  — a 1-L bag of normal saline via a giving set
  — the central venous catheter via extension tubing pre-flushed with the normal saline (to prevent air embolism)
  — a manometer clamped to a drip stand (Fig. 11.13).

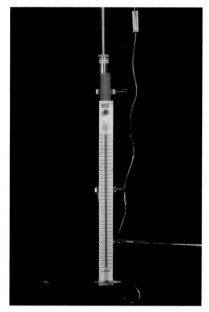

Fig. 11.13 The manometer clamped to a drip stand and attached via a 3-way tap to a bag of fluids (via a giving set, right-hand side) and the patient (via connecting tubing, left-hand side).

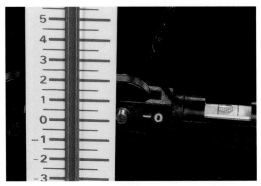

Fig. 11.14 Use the spirit level to ensure that the '0' reading on the manometer is directly level with a mark at the fourth intercostal space on the mid-axillary line.

- The patient should ideally be positioned in the supine recumbent position. If not possible, position the patient in a semi-recumbent position to a maximum angle of 45 degrees.
- The baseline point of reference of the manometer is 0. This must correspond with the level of the right atrium, which is taken as the fourth intercostal space in the mid-axillary line (preferably with the patient supine). Mark this point on the patient with a skin pen (to obtain accurate serial CVP measurements).
- Loosen the clamp on the manometer and slide the manometer until the '0' reading is level with the mark at the fourth intercostal space in the mid-axillary line. Tighten the clamp on the manometer in place on the drip stand at this point. Use the spirit level to ensure that the '0' reading on the manometer is directly in line with this mark on the patient (Fig. 11.14).
- Turn the 3-way tap off to the patient, allowing the manometer to fill with fluid.
- Once nearly full, turn the 3-way tap off to the intravenous fluid. The fluid level in the manometer will now fall until it levels off at the point of the patient's CVP (measured in cmH$_2$O, Fig. 11.15). The fluid level will oscillate at this point with the patient's ventilatory efforts, and the average reading between inspiration and expiration is taken as the CVP.
- Record serial CVP readings on a chart.
- Turn the 3-way tap off to the manometer and adjust the intravenous fluid infusion rate on the giving set.

SECTION 2 **Circulation**

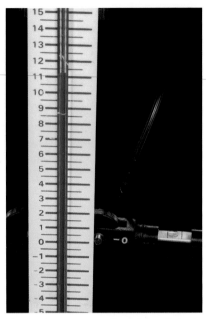

Fig. 11.15 The fluid level in the manometer will now fall until it levels off at the point of the patient's CVP (seen here to be just over 11 cmH$_2$O).

POST-PROCEDURE INVESTIGATIONS

- Always zero the CVP manometer to the point marked on the patient prior to taking a reading.
- It is the trend of serial CVP measurements that is useful in guiding volume status rather than the discrete CVP reading obtained.
- It should be remembered that CVP measurements are limited by the patient's co-morbidities, especially those giving rise to raised pulmonary arterial pressures.
- CVP measurements represent a diagnostic tool to be used *in addition* to clinical examination in the assessment of volume status.

SUGGESTED READING

NICE guidance. Central venous catheters – ultrasound locating devices.
Available online at:
http://www.nice.org.uk/Guidance/TA49

ARTERIAL BLOOD GAS SAMPLING

Gustav Magnus (1802–1870) made the first consistent analyses of blood gases in 1837. He obtained his blood samples from both horses and 'commoners who for a small sum permitted themselves to be bled'. Magnus went on to estimate the oxygen capacity of blood in 1845. However, modern blood gas analysis is the accumulation of the work of numerous brilliant men, namely Cremer (1865–1935), Haber (1868–1934), Hasselbalch (1874–1962), Van Slyke (1883–1971), Henderson (1878–1942), Astrup (1915–2000), Clark (1918–2005) and Severinghaus (1922–). These men pioneered the construction and refinement of the hydrogen, oxygen and carbon dioxide electrodes. Furthermore, they also constructed formulae to explain the relationships between the directly measured values of haemoglobin, oxygen tension, acidity and carbon dioxide, and the derived calculations of base deficit and bicarbonate.

INTRODUCTION

Arterial blood gas sampling provides useful information in the assessment of both respiratory function and acid–base balance. The usual site of puncture is the radial artery, although femoral and brachial arteries are common alternatives when the radial approach proves to be difficult. It is important to understand the anatomy of vessels in the area (Fig. 12.1) prior to puncture to ensure successful sampling, and to minimize discomfort and complications to the patient.

INDICATIONS

- Measurement of blood oxygen tension.
- Measurement of blood carbon dioxide tension.

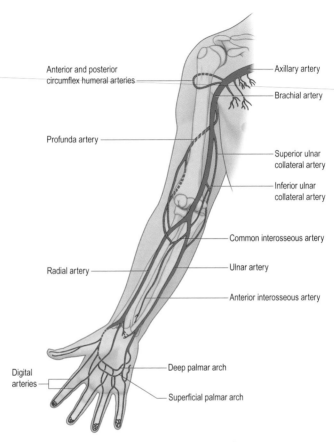

Anterior and posterior circumflex humeral arteries

Axillary artery

Brachial artery

Profunda artery

Superior ulnar collateral artery

Inferior ulnar collateral artery

Common interosseous artery

Radial artery

Ulnar artery

Anterior interosseous artery

Digital arteries

Deep palmar arch

Superficial palmar arch

Fig. 12.1   Anatomy of the collateral arterial supply to the hand.

- Measurement of acidaemia/alkalaemia (pH).
- Measurement of bicarbonate and base excess.

CONTRAINDICATIONS

- Local infection around predicted puncture site.
- Lack of consent.
- Negative Allen's test.

ALLEN'S TEST

Allen's test helps to ensure that while you are performing a radial puncture, the ulnar artery is capable of perfusing the hand. Ask the patient to clench a fist. Obstruct the radial and ulnar arteries using the index and second finger of both your hands on the respective arteries simultaneously. This prevents arterial flow into the hand. Ask the patient to open their hand while you are still occluding both arteries. Now release the pressure on the ulnar artery while still occluding the radial artery. This allows the ulnar artery blood to flow into the hand. Look for a change in colour from white to pink of all digits of the hand. This demonstrates that blood flow to the hand would be adequate should cannulation of the radial artery lead to its obstruction. This positive Allen's test is a prerequisite to radial cannulation and is a necessary precaution prior to puncture for gases. A negative Allen's test is a warning that digital ischaemia is a significant risk following radial artery cannulation for any period of time.

Research exists both in favour and against the reliability of Allen's test as a potential marker of ischaemic damage to the hand. You may wish to consider exploring the collateral circulation of the hand more definitively using a Doppler probe.

EQUIPMENT

- Pre-heparinized arterial blood gas sampling tube.
- Blue or green needle.
- Sterile alcohol swab.
- Cotton wool balls.
- Gloves.

PRACTICAL PROCEDURE

- Obtain consent.
- Ensure the patient is comfortable with their wrist supinated and held in a slightly extended position (if required, place the wrist over a pillow to aid dorsiflexion).
- Assemble the needle to a pre-heparinized syringe.

Tip Box

Unless you are very good at this procedure it is always kinder to inject some intradermal and subcutaneous lidocaine prior to obtaining a sample from the radial artery. It is always difficult to repeat procedures on patients who you have already hurt and failed on. They lose confidence in you, become tense and therefore hold their hand in a more flexed manner than ideal and at the point of puncture are more likely to withdraw their arm. The local anaesthetic wheal can be readily dispersed by rubbing the area prior to puncture.

SECTION 2   **Circulation**

- Wash your hands and wear gloves.
- Palpate for the radial arterial pulse and clean the area of skin with sterile alcohol swabs.
- Expel all of the heparin from the tube.
- Palpate for the radial arterial pulse along its length using two fingers. Warn the patient of a sharp scratch and puncture the skin at a 30–45 degree angle.
- Slowly advance the needle in the direction of the pulse until you get flashback (Fig. 12.2). Depending upon the make, the syringe either self-fills or the operator is required to pull on the plunger.

Tip Box

If you hit bone gently withdraw the needle while keeping its tip under the skin and proceed in a different direction of insertion.

- Once the sample has been taken, gently remove the needle and immediately apply firm pressure with the cotton wool ball to the site of needle insertion for 3–5 minutes.
- Remove the needle from the syringe. Gently tap the syringe in the upright position to allow air and air bubbles to rise to the top of the sample. Attach the air-filter bung and expel the air.
- Take immediately to an arterial blood gas sampling machine for analysis.

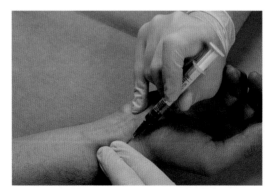

Fig. 12.2 Flashback of blood upon radial artery puncture.

FEMORAL ARTERY PUNCTURE

- Clean the area with antiseptic solution and feel for the femoral pulse. The femoral artery lies at the midpoint between the anterior superior iliac spine and the pubic symphysis (see Fig. 6.5), with the femoral nerve laterally and the femoral vein medially.
- Use a 21 G needle and insert at a 90 degree angle at the site of pulsation and proceed as above, remembering to apply firm pressure on the femoral artery for 5 minutes on removal of the needle.

Tip Box

Arterial blood gases may be difficult to obtain. The majority of the data from an arterial sample can be obtained from a central venous blood gas. For all intents and purposes venous base deficit, carbon dioxide tension (about 0.5 kPa higher) and pH (very slightly more acidic) are the same as arterial. Furthermore, while venous oxygenation (normally approximately 5.3 kPa) and saturation (normally approximately 75%) are considerably lower than corresponding arterial values, oxygen saturations measured by pulse oximetry when combined with a venous blood gas (in the absence of an arterial sample) would be more than adequate upon which to base acid–base or ventilatory clinical decisions. It is more important to obtain approximate information than abandon obtaining any information because it is not arterial.

- In extreme circumstances when attempts at arterial or venous sampling have failed, capillary samples from an ear lobe that has been rubbed provide very similar carbon dioxide, pH and bicarbonate measurements as an arterial sample.
- If you are struggling, get help!

COMPLICATIONS

- Pain.
- Failure to gain arterial sample: go to another site or ask for help.
- The sample obtained is in fact venous. If it is from the femoral or brachial you could use the information in conjunction with measuring pulse oximetry to indicate the adequacy of oxygenation.
- Bleeding.
- Haematoma formation.
- Infection at puncture site.
- Ischaemia of hand or finger due to emboli, spasm, aneurysm formation or thrombosis.

SECTION 2 **Circulation**

ARTERIAL CANNULATION

The Reverend Stephen Hales (1677–1761), a British veterinarian, cannulated the femoral artery of a horse using a brass tube and published his findings in 1733 in *Hemastatiks*. He connected the brass tube to a glass tube and recorded the rise of the blood column, thus becoming the first individual to measure blood pressure. This invasive approach was refined by Carl Ludwig in 1847 with his kymograph, which with the use of a quill plotted the waveform undulation of the arterial pulse. Non-invasive measurement followed individual observations and instrumental modifications by Karl Vierordt in 1855, Etienne Jules Mary in 1860, Samuel Von Basch in 1881 and Scipione Riva Rocci in 1896, cumulating into the modern day sphygmomanometer.

INTRODUCTION

Arterial cannulation is an advanced procedure performed on patients who require regular measurements of blood gases or who require continuous monitoring of blood pressure. It is normally performed on patients in a critical care environment. The radial artery is usually the vessel most suitable for cannulation. It is readily palpable and accessible, and the hand usually has an extensive collateral ulnar arterial circulation, thereby minimizing risk of digital ischaemia.

There are various cannulae available for arterial cannulation: some are the same design as venous cannulae whilst others are inserted using a guidewire approach. Note that whichever cannula is used it is unusual to use one larger than 20 G – larger cannulae risk damage to the vessel, whilst smaller cannulae become easily damped, kinked and provide poorer arterial traces. This chapter will concentrate on the insertion of guidewire-placed arterial cannulae using the Seldinger technique.

INDICATIONS

- Regular monitoring of arterial blood gases.
- Continuous or regular monitoring of blood pressure – mandatory if on inotropic support in the critical care setting.
- Patients undergoing major surgery, such as cardiovascular, cardiothoracic or neurosurgical procedures.

CONTRAINDICATIONS

- Negative Allen's test (see Chapter 12).
- Previous injury – such as from trauma, burns or surgery performed on the arm.
- Previous radial artery harvesting for coronary artery bypass surgery (may only have one vessel remaining for perfusion of the hand).
- Congenital deformities (such as in radial club hand) may result in anomalous vasculature to the extremity.
- A history of diabetes, hypertension, peripheral vascular disease, active infection in the extremity, collagen vascular disorders and blood dyscrasias may affect the decision to place the arterial catheter. All of these conditions have been associated with an increased risk of complications with arterial cannulation.
- Anticoagulant medications such as warfarin, aspirin, heparin and clopidogrel increase the risk of bleeding. This may lead to haematoma formation and a risk of hand ischaemia.
- Lack of consent.

EQUIPMENT

- 10 mL syringe.
- Green needle.
- Orange needle.
- Lidocaine.
- Dressing pack.
- Sterile gloves.
- Chlorhexidine cleaning solution.
- Heparin.
- Arterial cannula with guidewire and introducer needle (or 20 G simple arterial cannula).
- Gauze.
- Sutures and cutting blade.
- Clear sterile dressing.
- Transducer.

Tip Box

Ask a nurse to set up the transducer system and prepare a syringe of normal or heparinized saline prior to commencing the procedure. This should be ready to attach to the end of the cannula immediately on insertion.

NATIONAL PATIENT SAFETY AGENCY (NPSA) RECOMMENDATIONS

The NPSA recommends the use of 0.9% normal saline as a flush to maintain arterial line patency, with heparinized saline also permitted as a flush solution. However, it was also noted that the evidence base for using heparinized saline rather than normal saline as a flush for arterial lines is inconclusive (from the NHS National Electronic Library for Medicines, NELM). The NPSA report goes on to state that solutions used to flush arterial lines must not contain glucose.

PRACTICAL PROCEDURE

Tip Box

Ask the hand dominance of the patient and attempt to use the contralateral radial artery if possible.

- Obtain consent.
- Position the patient's wrist dorsiflexed over a pillow.
- Perform Allen's test (see Chapter 12) to confirm collateral circulation.
- Open the dressing pack and assemble equipment.
- Wash your hands and wear gloves.
- Clean the proposed site of entry over the radial artery.
- Draw up local anaesthetic into a 10 mL syringe with a green needle.
- Infiltrate intradermal and subcutaneous local anaesthetic around the presumed entry site with the orange needle. The local anaesthetic wheal can be readily dispersed by rubbing the area prior to puncture.
- Gently palpate the radial artery.
- Warn the patient of a sharp scratch.
- Hold the arterial needle at a 30 degree angle and insert with bevel upwards into the artery (Fig. 13.1). A 'give' is sometimes sensed followed by brisk blood flow, which should be pulsatile.

SECTION 2   **Circulation**

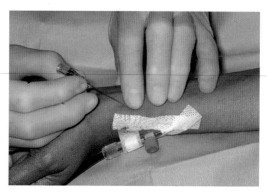

Fig. 13.1 Insert the arterial needle bevel upwards at a 30 degree angle.

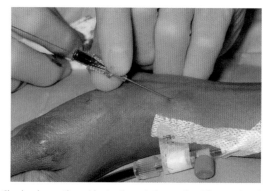

Fig. 13.2 Slowly advance the guidewire through the needle whilst ensuring that the wire remains in sight at all times from the free end.

- Slowly advance the guidewire through the needle and hence into the artery, allowing a portion of the guidewire to remain in sight *at all times* at the free end (Fig. 13.2).
- Remove the needle over the guidewire.
- Advance the arterial cannula over the wire making sure that the free end of the guidewire is obtained from the cannula prior to the cannula touching the skin (Fig. 13.3).
- Whilst holding the free end of the guidewire, slide the arterial cannula over the guidewire into the artery.
- Remove the guidewire.

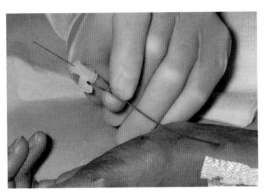

Fig. 13.3   Ensure that the free end of the guidewire has passed through the arterial line prior to the cannula touching the skin.

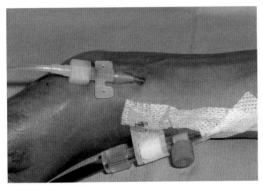

Fig. 13.4   Connect the transducer system and flush the arterial cannula.

- Connect the transducer system and flush the arterial cannula to ensure free flow (Fig. 13.4). A continuous arterial waveform and blood pressure should be evident with the transducer connected to the bedside monitor.

Tip Box

Ensure that the transducer is at the level of the patient's heart or the blood pressure readings will consequently be inaccurate.

SECTION 2   Circulation

- Suture the arterial line to the skin via the holes on the wings of the cannula.
- Apply a clear sterile dressing.
- Document the procedure clearly in the patient's medical notes.

Tip Box

If there are contraindications to using the radial artery, consider other vessels for cannulation. These may include the opposite radial artery, the femoral, ulnar or brachial arteries. Occasionally the dorsal artery of the foot, axillary and temporal arteries have been used.

POST-PROCEDURE INVESTIGATIONS

- Continuous transduction of the arterial waveform and blood pressure.
- Arterial blood gas sampling and analysis.

COMPLICATIONS

Despite constituting an invasive procedure, the risk of serious complications is less than 0.2%.

- Inadvertent disconnection when connections are manipulated, or accidental removal when the patient's position changes – both can cause significant unnoticed bleeding.
- Arterial thrombosis: increased risk in first 24 hours and with decreasing wrist circumference. This may require surgery to remove the clot or to bypass the artery, or thrombolytic therapy.

Tip Box

In the event of distal ischaemia, non-invasive arterial duplex ultrasonography can be done at the bedside to delineate areas of occlusion and flow through the artery. Angiography to evaluate the extent of injury to the radial artery may also be considered.

- Haematoma formation.
- Haemorrhage.
- Local infection of skin/subcutaneous tissue.
- Acute carpal tunnel syndrome.
- Compartment syndrome.
- Arterial aneurysm formation.

- Nerve injury.
- Ischaemia and skin/tissue necrosis.
- Air embolization – occurring with vigorous flushing of radial lines.
- Kinking of the line rendering it non-functional, particularly if the line is frequently redressed and remains hidden by dressings.

SUGGESTED READING

NPSA. Problems with infusions and sampling from arterial lines. Available online at: http://www.npsa.nhs.uk/patientsafety/alerts-and-directives/rapidrr/arterial-lines/

PERFORMING AN ELECTROCARDIOGRAM (ECG)

Augustus Desiré Waller (1856–1922), working at St Mary's Hospital in Paddington, London, produced the first electrocardiogram (ECG) recording in a human subject in 1887 using a Lippmann capillary electrometer attached to a projector. This projected the resultant trace onto a photographic plate that was moved by a toy train. Interestingly he saw little practical application for this, and it was not until Willem Einthoven (1860–1927) in Leiden used a string galvanometer rather than a capillary electrometer, which increased sensitivity, that the ECG became more usable. Einthoven went on to describe the tracing in terms of P, Q, R, S and T waves, and associated changes with some cardiac disorders. He was eventually rewarded with a Nobel Prize in 1924.

INTRODUCTION

The ECG is the basic investigation for diagnosing acute cardiac disorders. This procedure is normally undertaken by nursing staff but you need to be familiar with the process since positioning of the electrode leads will affect the accuracy of the ECG obtained.

INDICATIONS

- Suspected or confirmed acute coronary syndrome.
- Chest pain (of any nature).
- Shortness of breath (of any nature).
- Suspected arrhythmias.
- Collapse.
- Palpitations.

- Electrolyte abnormalities (particularly potassium).
- Suspected or confirmed bacterial endocarditis (to monitor for progressive lengthening of the PR interval).
- Pre-operative work-up.

EQUIPMENT

- 12-lead ECG machine.
- ECG leads – 4 limb leads and 6 chest leads.
- ECG lead attachment stickers.
- Razor.

PRACTICAL PROCEDURE

- Gain consent from the patient (to perform the ECG and the shaving of chest hair that this may entail).
- Place ECG lead attachment stickers for the limb leads to bony prominences at the wrists and just above the ankles (to reduce interference from skeletal muscle impulses) and attach the leads as in Table 14.1.

Tip Box

If the ECG stickers are not attaching to the patient, wipe away any sweat or body moisturizer.

- Shave the areas of the chest required for chest lead placement outlined below (Fig. 14.1). This ensures good sticker contact. Place ECG lead attachment stickers at these positions and attach the chest leads to the corresponding stickers.

TABLE 14.1 ECG limb lead placement

Limb lead	Colour of limb lead wire
Right wrist	RED
Left wrist	YELLOW
Right ankle	BLACK
Left ankle	GREEN

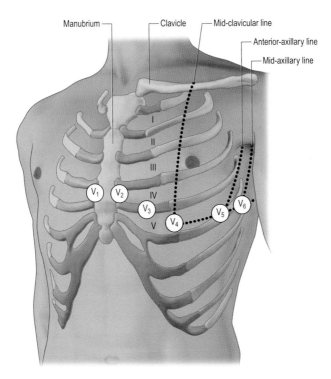

V_1	4th intercostal space, right sternal edge
V_2	4th intercostal space, left sternal edge
V_3	Mid-way (both horizontally and vertically) between V_2 and V_4
V_4	5th intercostal space, mid-clavicular line
V_5	Left anterior axillary line, horizontally aligned with V_4
V_6	Left mid-axillary line, horizontally aligned with V_4 and V_5

Fig. 14.1 Place lead-attachment stickers at these positions for the chest leads.

- Ensure that the ECG machine contains standard ECG graph paper and switch the machine on. Enter the patient's details.
- Make sure that the 'FILTER' button is on and that the machine is calibrated by pressing the 1 mV marker button. The height of the reference pulse mark on the resulting ECG will be 10 small squares.
- Ask the patient to relax, lie still and remain silent. Now acquire the ECG.
- Standard ECG paper speed runs at 25 mm/second. Each small square of the ECG measures 1 mm, which at 25 mm/second represents 0.04 seconds (Fig. 14.2).

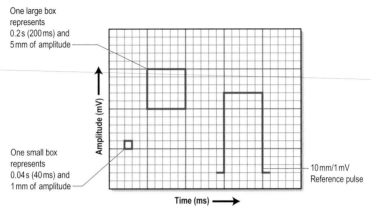

One large box represents 0.2 s (200 ms) and 5 mm of amplitude

Amplitude (mV)

One small box represents 0.04 s (40 ms) and 1 mm of amplitude

10 mm/1 mV Reference pulse

Time (ms) ⟶

Fig. 14.2 ECG graph paper measurements.

Five small squares constitute 1 large square, representing 0.2 seconds. Hence 1 second equates to 5 large squares.

- The calibration of the ECG voltage amplitude is set at 1 mV per 10 mm (i.e. the trace deflects 2 large squares vertically for every 1 mV signal detected).

Tip Box
- Other than a shivering patient, baseline interference or poor traces are invariably due to the poor sticker contact or faulty wiring. If after changing the stickers a problem persists, change the whole lead set.
- If the ECG reports an abnormal axis, check you have the limb leads correctly placed.

POST-PROCEDURE INVESTIGATIONS

- Date, time and add a patient label to the finished ECG.
- Note on the ECG if it was taken when the patient was experiencing symptoms (e.g. chest pain). This is of importance in the clinical interpretation of the ECG.

NASOGASTRIC TUBE PLACEMENT

The modern nasogastric (NG) tube is a 1921 modification by John Alfred Ryle (1889–1950). He covered the tip of the NG tube with rubber to prevent injury to the gastric mucosa, unlike previous tubes which had a metal bulb at their tip. However, the earliest recording of using a tube for enteral nutrition was that of the Seville-born Arab surgeon Ibn Zuhr (also known as Avenzoar, 1091–1161) who fed a patient with an oesophageal stricture via a silver tube. Incidentally Ibn Zuhr is also credited with the first correct description of performing a tracheotomy for suffocating patients.

INTRODUCTION

Nasogastric tube placement is a simple procedure, but can be unpleasant for the conscious patient. This is commonly performed by nursing staff; however, junior doctors would be expected to place them if these initial attempts are unsuccessful. Small-diameter (8–12 Fr) tubes are frequently used for patents who require enteral feeding. Larger tubes (14 Fr or larger) are used to administer medications, provide gastric decompression or allow continuous aspiration of retained gastric contents. These larger tubes are acceptable for feeding over a short period, usually less than 1 week. Small-bore NG tubes cause less trauma to the nasal mucosa both during insertion and while in situ, and are better tolerated. Placement errors lead to potentially major complications, most commonly when mistakenly placed in the respiratory tract. Failure to observe pathological states that constitute a contraindication to NG tube placement can result in passage of the tube into the brain (base of skull fracture) or peritoneum (upper GI perforation).

INDICATIONS

WIDE-BORE NASOGASTRIC TUBES

- Bowel obstruction.
- Gastric outlet obstruction.

FINE-BORE NASOGASTRIC TUBES

- Enteric feeding.

CONTRAINDICATIONS

- Coagulopathy (a relative contraindication).
- Oesophageal varices.
- Maxillofacial and oropharyngeal trauma or surgery.
- Skull fractures.
- Unstable cervical spine injury.
- Laryngectomy.
- Compromised airway.

EQUIPMENT

- Sterile gloves.
- Kidney bowl.
- Gauze.
- Lubricant jelly.
- NG tube.
- 10 mL syringe.
- Litmus paper.
- Medical adhesive tape.
- Drainage bag.
- Gloves.
- Glass of water with straw.

PRACTICAL PROCEDURE

- Explain the procedure to the patient and obtain consent.
- Wash your hands and wear sterile gloves.
- Ensure that the end of the NG tube will fit the drainage bag to be used.

- The patient should be in an upright position, the head supported with pillows if needed to ensure that it is not tilting backwards.
- Check the patency of the nostrils; ask the patient to blow their nose if needed.
- Lubricate the NG tube tip and the first 10 cm.
- Slowly insert the NG tube into a nostril using a rotating motion and advance it horizontally along the base of the nasal cavity until it reaches the posterior pharynx (and hence usually induces the gag reflex).

Tip Box

When the NG tube is in the pharynx, rotate the tube 180 degrees to encourage passage of the tube into the oesophagus rather than the trachea. This is especially useful if the tube has been refrigerated, making it more rigid.

Tip Box

If you are having trouble passing the NG tube, try asking the patient to put their chin to their chest and insert the tube as above until it reaches the posterior pharynx.

Tip Box

If you are experiencing trouble passing the tube into the oesophagus because it is too soft and it keeps folding on itself in the back of the throat, try putting the tube in the fridge for 20 minutes for it to harden, or consider a larger tube.

- Ask the patient to swallow water repeatedly through a straw whilst advancing the NG tube during the swallow. In this manner the patient effectively swallows the tube into the oesophagus.
- Advance the NG tube down the oesophagus and into the stomach (Fig. 15.1). The NG tube is graduated every 10 cm (usual mouth to stomach distance is 35–40 cm). Hence insert the NG tube to the 40 cm mark.
- Ensure the NG tube is sitting in the stomach:
  — Gently aspirate stomach contents with a syringe and test with litmus paper (if in the stomach the pH should be less than 4). Remember, patients on proton pump

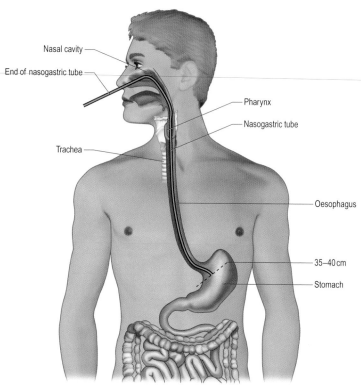

Nasal cavity

End of nasogastric tube

Pharynx

Nasogastric tube

Trachea

Oesophagus

35–40 cm

Stomach

Fig. 15.1 Insert the nasogastric tube to 40 cm as a guide to siting the tip in the stomach.

inhibitors, antacids and H_2 antagonists may have a high gastric pH and hence aspiration tests may not be accurate. X-ray confirmation may have to be used in these patients.

— Small-bore NG tubes commonly do not allow aspiration of stomach contents and require chest X-ray confirmation of position.

— If you are unable to get adequate stomach contents to test for pH, the patient will need to have a chest X-ray to check the position of the tube. The tip of the tube must be seen to be below the diaphragm.

• Attach the drainage bag.

• Secure the NG tube around the patient's nose with micropore tape taking care not to exert too much pressure on the nares adjacent to the NG tube.

• Document the date and time of NG tube insertion. Document the type of tube inserted, the batch number, any complications or difficulties in insertion and how the correct position of the tube was confirmed.

POST-PROCEDURE INVESTIGATIONS

- If you are in any way unsure about the position of the NG tube, obtain a chest X-ray. The NG tube tip has a radio opaque line at the end and can therefore be seen. However, this X-ray confirmation is valid only at the time of the X-ray.
- The NG tube should not be used until positive evidence of its placement has been obtained (pH or chest X-ray).
- Syringing air down the NG tube whist auscultating the epigastrium is an unreliable method of checking tube position due to transmitted lung sounds.

COMPLICATIONS

- Failure to pass the NG tube.
- Epistaxis.
- NG tube passed into trachea.
- Oesophageal, pharyngeal or gastric perforation.
- NG tube in duodenum – should this be confirmed on chest X-ray pull the tube back approximately 5 cm.
- Oesophagitis and stricture formation secondary to oesophageal inflammation.
- Retropharyngeal or nasopharyngeal necrosis.
- Sinusitis from NG tube in situ for a prolonged period of time.

CHAPTER 16

ABDOMINAL PARACENTESIS AND ASCITIC DRAIN INSERTION

Hippocrates (460–377 BC) was known to have utilized abdominal paracentesis for the treatment of ascites. Accumulated abdominal fluid was frequently the endpoint of congestive cardiac failure. One of the earliest treatments for fluid accumulation (hydropsy or dropsy) involved use of fine percutaneous tubes to cause seepage of interstitial fluid. These famous Herbert Southey's (1783–1865) silver tubes were used for any oedematous part of the body. A natural extension of such therapy was abdominal paracentesis. Ludwig van Beethoven (1770–1827) underwent repeated paracentesis for ascites related to cirrhosis (undiagnosed at the time). Historians have recently blamed Beethoven's doctor for contributing to his death by lead poisoning due to the poultices applied to the paracentesis sites!

ABDOMINAL PARACENTESIS

INTRODUCTION

Abdominal paracentesis is performed as a supplementary diagnostic procedure to determine the cause of ascites or new abdominal pain in patients with ascites. In cirrhotic patients it is commonly performed when there is a suspicion that new symptomatology is due to spontaneous bacterial peritonitis or malignancy. Coagulopathies are not contraindications to the procedure given a large number of patients with ascites of hepatic origin will have abnormal clotting. Ascitic paracentesis has been outlined below in accordance with the British Society of Gastroenterology guidelines.

INDICATIONS

- Diagnostic investigations of abdominal ascites.

CONTRAINDICATIONS

- Local infection overlying the puncture site.
- Highly deranged coagulopathy.
- Lack of consent.

EQUIPMENT

- Dressing pack.
- Sterile gloves.
- Orange needle.
- Green needle × 2.
- 20 mL syringe.
- 10 mL syringe.
- Lidocaine.
- Gauze.
- Chlorhexidine cleaning solution.
- Sterile drapes.
- Plaster.
- Skin pen.
- Blood culture bottles.
- Blood glucose tube–fluoride oxalate tube.
- EDTA tube.
- Sterile bottles × 2.

PRACTICAL PROCEDURE

- Explain the procedure to the patient and gain consent.
- If ascites is not distending the abdomen it is prudent to undertake ultrasound examination to locate the fluid.

Tip Box

Ensure the patient has an empty bladder prior to the procedure.

- Position the patient in a supine position on a bed. Ask them to move towards your side of the bed and place a pillow under their head for comfort.

- Raise the level of the bed until their abdomen is at a comfortable height for you to perform the procedure.
- Palpate and percuss the edge of the liver to ensure you know its position.
- Percuss the ascites by assessing for shifting dullness: percuss the abdomen in the supine position listening for the transition point between resonance and dullness. The central abdomen should be resonant and the flanks dulled by the presence of dependent ascites. Ask the patient to then roll into the lateral position and wait approximately 5 seconds. Percuss over the area that was previously dull: if this now sounds resonant, this is indicative of shifting dullness.
- A spot lateral to this in the right or left lower quadrant can be marked but should be in the safe area (Fig. 16.1A and B). The commonest site for an ascitic tap is about 15 cm lateral to the umbilicus in the left or right lower quadrant. The aim is to avoid solid structures such as liver and spleen in the upper abdomen and the lower epigastric arteries and bowel in the lower abdomen.

Tip Box
Avoid areas with superficial dilated veins, especially in the presence of portal hypertension.

- Wash your hands and wear sterile gloves.
- Clean the area and place the sterile drapes.
- Draw up the lidocaine in a 10 mL syringe and attach the orange needle.
- Warn the patient of a sharp scratch and infiltrate 2 mL of the local anaesthetic subcutaneously over the marked area using an orange needle.
- Check the area is adequately anaesthetized with gentle poking of the skin with the needle.
- Infiltrate local anaesthetic into deeper tissues advancing the green needle obliquely until ascitic fluid is aspirated.

Tip Box
This oblique direction is termed the 'Z track', ensuring the sites of needle entry at the skin and at the peritoneum do not overlie one another. This reduces the risk of continuing leak from the puncture site following the procedure.

- Assemble the 20 mL syringe and green needle.
- At the same puncture site slowly insert the green needle and advance it along the anaesthetized track whilst continually aspirating.

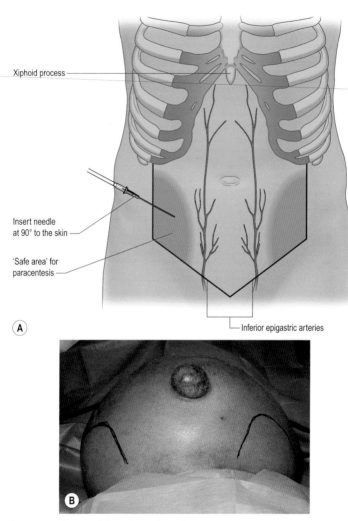

Xiphoid process

Insert needle
at 90° to the skin

'Safe area' for
paracentesis

Ⓐ

Inferior epigastric arteries

Ⓑ

Fig. 16.1 'Safe area' of the abdomen for performing paracentesis: the right or left iliac
fossae inferior to the umbilicus. (A) Line drawing of the surface anatomy of the abdomen
for safe abdominal paracentesis. (B) Photo demonstrating the safe areas for paracentesis
in a patient with gross ascites.

- Once the required volume of the sample has been obtained, withdraw the needle and place firm pressure on the area with some gauze.
- Apply a sterile dressing.
- Inoculate ascitic fluid into blood culture bottles, specimen bottles, a fluoride-oxalate tube and an EDTA tube.
- Document the procedure clearly in the patient's medical notes. Note the macroscopic appearance of the fluid (e.g. straw-coloured, turbid, haemorrhagic).
- Advise the patient to lie on the opposite side to paracentesis for approximately 2 hours should any ascites leak from the site of aspiration.

POST-PROCEDURE INVESTIGATIONS

- Cell count – particularly looking at the neutrophil count (>250 white cells/mm^3 is diagnostic of spontaneous bacterial peritonitis).
- Microscopy, culture and sensitivity including acid-fast bacilli.
- Cytology.
- Glucose.
- Lactate dehydrogenase (LDH).
- Amylase (increased in pancreatitis).
- Protein.
- Albumin (with concurrent serum albumin to determine the serum–ascites albumin gradient).
- Alpha-fetoprotein (AFP).
- pH.
- Gamma-glutamyl transpeptidase (increased in hepatoma).

COMPLICATIONS

Complications are uncommon. Approximately 1% of taps result in superficial abdominal haematomas, with intraperitoneal complications such as haemoperitoneum or bowel perforations occurring in less than 1 in 1000 taps. In the presence of bleeding diatheses (e.g. significant thrombocytopaenia or coagulopathy) it would be reasonable to perform the procedure under platelet or fresh frozen plasma (FFP) cover, respectively. However, there is little evidence that this reduces the risk of bleeding for this procedure.

- Pain.
- Infection around puncture site.
- Bacterial peritonitis.
- Bleeding around puncture site.
- Leaking of ascitic fluid around puncture site.
- Dry tap.
- Perforation of bowel wall or bladder.

Tip Box

In the case of a dry tap ask the patient to gently roll towards you so that the ascites accumulates at the site of aspiration. However, an abdominal ultrasound scan to mark the best site for paracentesis would be the investigation of choice in this setting.

ASCITIC DRAIN INSERTION

INTRODUCTION

Ascitic drain insertion is indicated for the relief of raised intra-abdominal pressure secondary to large-volume ascites. This may compromise urine output through reduced renal perfusion (intra-abdominal hypertension >30 cm water) or ventilatory function with increasing carbon dioxide tension.

Large-volume ascites commonly develops in portal hypertension due to primary liver disease, severe right heart failure or malignancy. The removal of large volume ascites secondary to liver cirrhosis necessitates simultaneous intravenous replacement with albumin as per British Society of Gastroenterology guidelines to maintain the intravascular volume in the face of large fluid shifts. The administration of albumin per se in liver disease, however, does not reduce the rate at which ascites reaccumulates; this is controlled by measures that reduce portal hypertension.

INDICATIONS

Relief of symptoms due to tense ascites:

- pain
- progressive oliguria secondary to intra-abdominal hypertension
- progressive ventilatory difficulty.

Tip Box

Whilst the release of purulent fluid from a collection to reduce bacterial load is common practice with abscesses (an empyema, for example), the British Society of Gastroenterology states that there is no available evidence to support this line of management in the case of spontaneous bacterial peritonitis (SBP). Therefore the role of total paracentesis in the management of SBP remains a matter of debate and varied practice, and local gastroenterology or hepatology advice and policy should be consulted prior to considering this measure.

CONTRAINDICATIONS

- Local infection overlying the puncture site.
- Highly deranged coagulopathy.
- Bowel obstruction.
- Lack of consent.

EQUIPMENT

- Dressing pack.
- Sterile gloves.
- Orange needle (25 G).
- Green needle (21 G).
- 1 × 10 mL syringe.
- 1 × 20 mL syringe.
- Lidocaine.
- Gauze.
- Chlorhexidine cleaning solution.
- Sterile drapes.
- Transparent sterile dressing.
- Suture.
- Suture cutter.
- Bonanno® catheter ascitic drain.
- Drainage bag.
- Skin pen.

PRACTICAL PROCEDURE

- Gain consent.

Tip Box

Ensure the patient has an empty bladder prior to the procedure.

- Position the patient in a supine position on a bed. Ask them to move towards your side of the bed and place a pillow under their head for comfort.
- Raise the level of the bed until their abdomen is at your height or just below.
- Palpate and percuss the edge of the liver to ensure you know its position.
- Percuss the ascites by assessing for shifting dullness: percuss the abdomen in the supine position listening for the transition point between resonance and dullness. Ideally the ascites should be assessed by ultrasound and the site of maximum ascitic depth marked by the radiologist. Mark the site for puncture in the safe area (see Fig. 16.1B).

Tip Box

Avoid areas with superficial dilated veins, especially in the presence of portal hypertension.

- Wash your hands and wear sterile gloves.
- Clean the area and place the sterile drapes.
- Draw up the local anaesthetic in a 10 ml syringe and attach the orange needle.
- Assemble the ascitic drain as instructed (Fig. 16.2).
- Warn the patient of a sharp scratch and infiltrate 1 mL of the local anaesthetic subcutaneously over the marked area.
- Check the area is adequately anaesthetized with gentle poking of the skin with the needle.
- Infiltrate local anaesthetic into deeper tissues with a green needle until ascitic fluid is aspirated (Fig. 16.3). While withdrawing the needle, line the track with local anaesthetic.

Tip Box

When siting an ascitic drain in patients with peritoneal metastases use up to 10 mL lidocaine. If you hit peritoneal deposits, gently withdraw the needle slightly and proceed in a different direction.

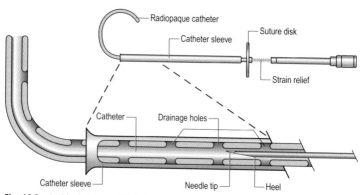

Fig. 16.2 Ascitic drain assembly (adapted from Bonanno® catheter instructions). With the catheter sleeve proximal to the suture disk, advance the trocar into the catheter bevel-down to the centre of the catheter sleeve. Subsequently advance the trocar (bevel-down) and the catheter sleeve simultaneously down the length of the catheter, maintaining the position of the trocar tip relative to the centre of the catheter sleeve. Once the bevel emerges from the catheter tip, screw the trocar in place into the catheter hub. Discard the catheter sleeve.

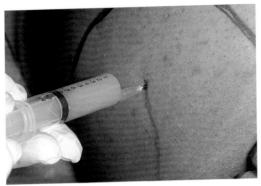

Fig. 16.3 Infiltrate local anaesthetic into deeper tissues with a green needle until ascitic fluid is aspirated.

Tip Box

Never attempt drain insertion if you have been unable to obtain ascitic aspirate at the time of local anaesthetic infiltration.

- Attach a 20 mL syringe to the assembled drain apparatus. Introduce the ascitic drain trocar at a 90 degree angle to the abdominal wall. Hold the apparatus with two hands using the hand closest to the abdominal wall to regulate the length of drain inserted, ensuring that only a small length of the drain apparatus is inserted at a time. This minimizes the potential trauma were the whole or most of the trocar to inadvertently enter the abdominal cavity. Advance the trocar slowly whilst aspirating the syringe until ascitic fluid is obtained (Fig. 16.4).
- Unscrew the locking mechanism between the trocar and the drain.
- Using your non-dominant hand gently slide the drain into the abdominal cavity over the trocar, and with your dominant hand subsequently withdraw the trocar out of the drain as you would a cannula (Fig. 16.5).

Tip Box

Ensure when withdrawing the trocar you do not withdraw it too quickly otherwise the drain will kink.

- Attach the drainage bag (Fig. 16.6).
- Suture the drain to skin through the preformed suture holes on the flange of the drain.

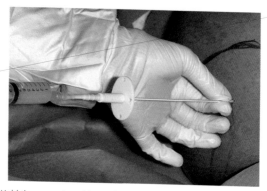

Fig. 16.4 Hold the apparatus with two hands to regulate the length of drain inserted. Advance slowly whilst aspirating the syringe until ascitic fluid is obtained.

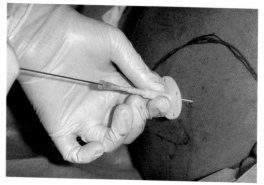

Fig. 16.5 Gently slide the drain into the abdominal cavity over the trocar, with the trocar held still (and subsequently removed) by your dominant hand as you would a cannula.

- Place a clear sterile dressing over the drain entry site.
- Document the procedure clearly in the patient's medical notes.

Tip Box

If attempts to insert a drain fail, the ascites may be loculated. Obtain an ultrasound-guided drain.

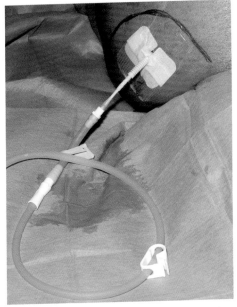

Fig. 16.6   Suture the drain in place via preformed suture holes on the flange of the drain and place a clear sterile dressing over the drain entry site.

POST-PROCEDURE CARE AND INVESTIGATIONS

- Send ascitic fluid for the same range of investigations as you would when performing a diagnostic tap (see under Abdominal paracentesis investigations section).
- Request post-procedure observations at regular intervals of approximately 15 minutes for the first hour, then hourly thereafter, in particular relating to the patient's volume status. Keep a strict fluid balance chart, noting the volume of ascites drained, the volume of intravenous fluid replacement (if required) and the urine output.

Tip Box

- The British Society of Gastroenterology guidelines for the management of ascites **secondary to cirrhosis** recommend:
  — An albumin infusion as a plasma expander when large volumes (i.e. greater than 5 L) are removed. For each litre of ascites removed infuse 8 g of albumin (i.e. 100 mL 20% albumin administered for every 3 L ascites drained).
  — A synthetic plasma expander may be used when less than 5 L of ascites has been removed.

- In the event of haemodynamic compromise consider intravenous volume expansion with a synthetic colloid plasma expander and hold off further drainage until haemodynamic stability is achieved.
- Aim to drain the ascites to dryness in a single session of not more than 1–4 hours. The ascitic drain should preferably be removed as soon as the original symptoms for placement of the drain have been controlled. Sterile ascitic fluid is at risk of becoming infected if drains are left in for more than 24 hours.

COMPLICATIONS

In the presence of bleeding diatheses (e.g. significant thrombocytopaenia or coagulopathy) it would be reasonable to perform the procedure under platelet or FFP cover, respectively. However, there is little evidence that this reduces the risk of bleeding for this procedure.

- Pain.
- Infection around puncture site.
- Bacterial peritonitis.
- Bleeding around drain site.
- Leaking of ascitic fluid around drain site – a suture (ideally a purse-string) may be used to close the drain track.
- Dry tap – obtain an ultrasound to look for loculated ascites.
- Hypotension.
- Perforation of bowel wall or bladder.

SUGGESTED READING

Moore KP, Aithal GP (2006) Guidelines on the management of ascites in cirrhosis. Gut, 55(suppl 6): vi1–vi12.
http://www.bsg.org.uk/pdf_word_docs/ascites_cirrhosis.pdf

RIGID SIGMOIDOSCOPY

The *Corpus Hippocraticum* of early medical works from ancient Greece described both proctoscopy and use of the rectal speculum, constituting the earliest published reference to endoscopy.

INTRODUCTION

Rigid sigmoidoscopy is a procedure that is usually performed in an out-patient setting. The transparent anoscope allows a 360 view of the anal canal and rectum, and hence has a significant role in the evaluation of anorectal and distal colonic pathology. This invasive procedure should be performed with care and sensitivity, maintaining the patient's dignity at all times. This can only be learned after observing a senior colleague perform the procedure, and subsequently talking through the technique before performing it yourself under supervision.

INDICATIONS

- Symptoms or signs suggestive of anorectal or colonic pathology.
- As a routine investigation prior to anorectal procedures.
- Biopsy of anal canal.
- Removal of foreign bodies in the anal canal.

CONTRAINDICATIONS

Some of these are relative contraindications. The main concern is that of potential perforation.

- Lack of consent.
- Confirmed or suspected perforation of the bowel.

- Toxic megacolon.
- Fulminant colitis.
- Severe diverticulitis.
- Peritonitis.

EQUIPMENT

- Gloves.
- Eye visor/goggles.
- Gauze swabs.
- Lubricant gel.
- Disposable rigid obturator assembled with the outer plastic anoscope (Fig. 17.1).
- Attachable non-disposable light-head (connected to mains) and bellows (Fig. 17.2).

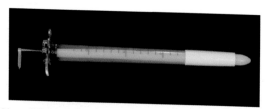

Fig. 17.1   Disposable rigid obturator assembled with the outer plastic anoscope.

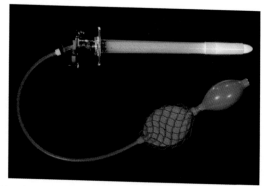

Fig. 17.2   Non-disposable light-head (connected to mains) and bellows attached to anoscope.

PRACTICAL PROCEDURE

Tip Box

The bowels should be emptied pre-procedure with a glycerine suppository or phosphate enema.

- Explain the procedure and obtain consent.
- Set up the equipment on a clean trolley.
- Plug the equipment into the light source to ensure that it functions correctly.
- Position the patient into the left lateral decubitus (Sims') position with the buttocks to the edge of the examination couch.
- Wash your hands, wear gloves and eye visor/goggles.
- Inspect the perineum and anus for evidence of fistulae, abscesses or skin tags.
- Go on to perform a digital rectal examination.
- Having completed the rectal examination, assemble the rigid obturator with the overlying plastic anoscope and apply lubricating gel.
- Attach the non-disposable light-head (connected to mains) and bellows.
- Gently insert the lubricated device approximately 5 cm into the anus in the direction of the navel.
- Remove the obturator (Fig. 17.3).
- Using the bellows of the rigid sigmoidoscope inflate a little air to open the anal canal and advance the sigmoidoscope further into the distal colon under direct vision up to 20 cm from the anal verge (Fig. 17.4).

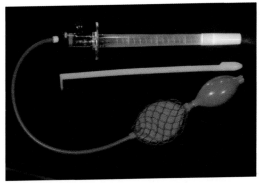

Fig. 17.3 Removal of the obturator allowing light to pass through the anoscope.

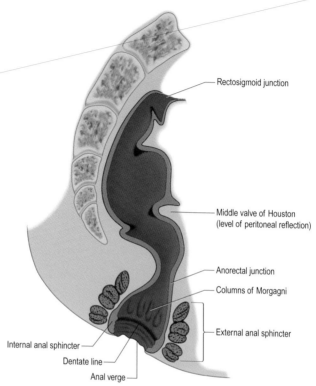

Rectosigmoid junction

Middle valve of Houston
(level of peritoneal reflection)

Anorectal junction

Columns of Morgagni

External anal sphincter

Internal anal sphincter

Dentate line

Anal verge

Fig. 17.4 Cross-section of anorectal anatomy.

- Having advanced to the required distance, slowly withdraw the rigid
  sigmoidoscope under direct vision, inspecting the bowel wall and the anal canal for
  fistulae openings, abscesses, fissures, internal haemorrhoids or neoplastic lesions.

Tip Box

If either the patient experiences pain in the Sims' position or you are unable
to gain good views, try altering their position. The jack-knife position is an
alternative that requires a special table that breaks in the middle (Fig. 17.5).
Position the patient in a prone position on the table and secure them to the
table with the straps. Lower the top of the table so the upper body and head
are tilting downwards.

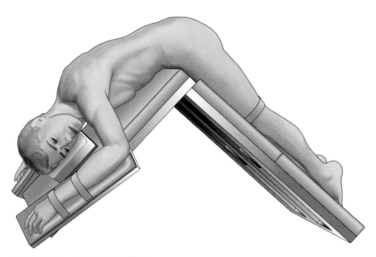

Fig. 17.5   The 'jack-knife' position.

COMPLICATIONS

- Pain: should this occur, stop and remove the anoscope.
- Perforation.
- Infection.
- Haemorrhage.
- Localized bleeding.

URETHRAL CATHETERIZATION

Sushruta, a surgeon of ancient India (circa 6th century BC), described gold, silver, iron and wood tubes lubricated with ghee for the evacuation of urine. Aulus Cornelius Celsus (25 BC–AD 50) described bronze and lead pipes for urethral catheterization in *De Re Medicina*. Frederick Foley, a medical student in Boston, designed the modern catheter in the 1930s. Fortunately catheters now come in latex, silicone, Teflon and PVC, with some coated in silver alloy to reduce catheter-related infection.

INTRODUCTION

Catheterization is an invasive procedure. It should be carried out in a sensitive manner, maintaining the patient's dignity at all times. The indication of catheterization determines whether long- or short-term catheters are used and should be considered prior to the procedure.

MALE CATHETERIZATION

INDICATIONS

- Acute urinary retention.
- Haematuria.
- Accurate assessment of urinary output (a measure of organ perfusion) and volume status (e.g. in circulatory shock or acute renal failure).
- Delivery of medications (e.g. warmed fluids in the treatment of hypothermia, chemotherapeutic agents in the treatment of bladder carcinoma).

Tip Box

A three-way catheter may be required if the indication is urinary retention due to clots (clot-retention). The same technique for catheter insertion as described above applies, with bladder irrigation being delivered via a third catheter lumen.

CONTRAINDICATIONS

- Lack of consent.
- Phimosis/paraphimosis (a relative contraindication).
- Urethral stricture.
- Penile fracture.

EQUIPMENT

- Dressing pack.
- Male catheter.
- Catheter drainage bag.
- Normal saline cleaning solution.
- Gauze.
- Sterile lidocaine anaesthetic gel (e.g. Instillagel®).
- 10 mL sterile water.
- 10 mL syringe.
- Sterile gloves.
- Disposable, loose-fitting outer sterile gloves.
- Kidney bowl.

CATHETER SIZE

Urethral catheters are measured in charrières (ch) after the 19th century French instrument maker Joseph Charrières, representing the outer diameter of the catheter. The size of the catheter in charrières is equivalent to three times its diameter in millimetres (mm): for example, a 12 ch catheter measures 4 mm in diameter. These measurements are commonly referred to as 'French gauge'. A larger-gauge catheter may be required in circumstances such as haematuria or pyuria, where clots or debris may obstruct urinary flow. In these cases a three-way catheter may be required, with bladder irrigation being delivered via a third catheter lumen to maintain catheter patency. Larger catheters are more likely to cause urethral damage, but too small a catheter can result in leakage around the catheter. Various types are available: Foley, Coude tip (elbow shaped at the tip for negotiating the prostate) and straight. The smallest Foley catheter likely to be effective is normally first choice for general use, usually size 10, 12 or 14 ch in adults.

Tip Box
If the catheter will not pass down the urethra (commonly due to an enlarged prostate or urethral stricture), consider using more anaesthetic gel and inserting a larger-sized catheter. Paradoxical though this may seem, a larger catheter will be less flexible in the urethra and hence more likely to negotiate the tighter prostatic urethra. However, never apply substantial force when inserting a catheter; if the catheter does not pass (secondary to a stricture, for example) withdraw the catheter and discuss with a urologist.

PRACTICAL PROCEDURE

See Fig. 18.1.

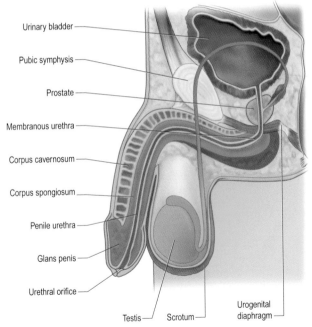

Fig. 18.1   Cross-section of male urogenital anatomy.

- Explain the procedure to the patient and gain consent.
- Open the equipment onto a clean trolley, ensuring the urinary catheter remains inside the internal packaging.

- Wash your hands and wear sterile gloves with a second overlying pair of disposable sterile gloves.
- Fill a syringe with 10 mL sterile water.
- Hold the penis with a sterile gauze swab around the shaft with your non-dominant hand.
- Retract the foreskin and gently cleanse the urethral meatus with gauze soaked in normal saline, directing the wiping motion away from the urethra.
- Place sterile drapes over the exposed groin and make a hole in the drape to place the penis through.
- Gently insert the pre-filled lidocaine gel syringe tip into the urethral meatus of the penis.
- Warn the patient of a stinging sensation and slowly insert 10 mL of the lidocaine gel.
- Dispose of the outer gloves.
- Expose the catheter tip from the inner packaging by tearing the perforations and gently insert the catheter into the urethral meatus with your dominant hand, holding it through its inner package.
- As you advance the catheter using a twisting or rotating motion continue to release it from its inner package by tearing the perforations, hence maintaining a 'non-touch technique'.
- Advance the full length of the catheter to its bifurcation and place a kidney bowl between the patient's legs.
- Remove the last of the inner packaging and attach the catheter bag.
- Once urine is draining, inflate the balloon with 10 mL of sterile water.
- Gently pull back the catheter until resistance is felt and it resumes a fixed position (i.e. the catheter balloon is at the bladder neck).
- Pull forward the penile foreskin (to prevent paraphimosis).
- Wipe off any excess lidocaine gel.
- The catheter bag should hang below pelvis level to avoid retrograde flow and catheter-borne infections.
- Record the date and time the catheter was inserted in the patient's medical notes. Note:
  — the type and size of catheter used
  — the volume of sterile water used to inflate the catheter balloon
  — the residual volume
  — post-procedure investigations and complications.

FEMALE CATHETERIZATION

INDICATIONS

- Acute retention of urine.
- Haematuria.
- Accurate assessment of urinary output (a measure of organ perfusion) and volume status (e.g. in circulatory shock or acute renal failure).
- Delivery of medications (e.g. warmed fluids in the treatment of hypothermia, chemotherapeutic agents in the treatment of bladder carcinoma).

CONTRAINDICATIONS

- Lack of consent.

EQUIPMENT

- Dressing pack.
- Female catheter.
- Catheter drainage bag.
- Normal saline cleaning solution.
- Gauze.
- Sterile lidocaine anaesthetic gel (e.g. Instillagel®).
- 10 mL sterile water.
- 10 mL syringe.
- Sterile gloves.
- Disposable, loose-fitting outer sterile gloves.
- Kidney bowl.

PRACTICAL PROCEDURE

See Fig. 18.2.

- Explain the procedure to the patient and gain consent.
- Position the patient supine on the bed with their legs bent and then relaxed open, exposing the perineum (take care when positioning patients with prosthetic hip or knee replacements). Ensure that the perineum is well lit (e.g. using a gynaecology bedside lamp).
- Open the equipment onto a clean trolley, ensuring the urinary catheter remains inside the internal packaging.
- Wash your hands and wear sterile gloves with a second overlying pair of disposable sterile gloves.
- Fill a syringe with 10 mL sterile water.
- Part the labia with the fingers of your non-dominant hand. Using your dominant hand gently cleanse the perineum with gauze soaked in sterile normal saline wiping from anterior to posterior (i.e. towards the anus to avoid introducing microbes from this region).
- Place sterile drapes over the groin leaving the perineum exposed.
- Dispose of the outer gloves.
- Expose the catheter tip from the inner packaging by tearing the perforations and apply 2–3 mL of lidocaine gel.
- Part the labia with the fingers of your non-dominant hand, and gently insert the catheter into the urethra with your dominant hand holding it through its inner package.
- As you advance the catheter continue to release it from its inner package by tearing the perforations, hence maintaining a 'non-touch technique'.
- Advance the full length of the catheter to its bifurcation and place a kidney bowl between the patient's legs.

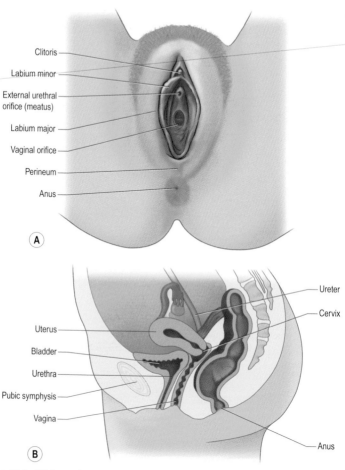

Fig. 18.2 (A) External anatomy of the female urogenital area. (B) Cross-section of female urogenital anatomy.

 Tip Box

If resistance is felt while attempting to advance the catheter, ask the patient to relax and take deep breaths or cough and slowly pass the catheter using a twisting or rotating motion. These manoeuvres aim to alleviate the perineal muscle spasm that commonly hinders passage of the urethral catheter.

- Remove the last of the inner packaging and attach the catheter bag.
- Once urine is draining, inflate the balloon with 10 mL of sterile water.
- Gently pull back the catheter until resistance is felt and it resumes a fixed position (i.e. the catheter balloon is at the bladder neck).
- Wipe away any excess lidocaine gel.
- The catheter bag should hang below pelvis level to avoid retrograde flow and catheter-borne infections.
- Record the date and time the catheter was inserted in the patient's medical notes. Note:
    — the type and size of catheter used
    — the volume of sterile water used to inflate the catheter balloon
    — the residual volume
    — post-procedure investigations and complications.

Tip Box
The absence of urine on inserting the catheter its full length to the bifurcation implies one of two possibilities: an empty bladder or insertion into a false passage. Try to flush the catheter with 50 mL of sterile normal saline using a bladder syringe. If this flushes easily and can subsequently be aspirated, it is most likely that the catheter tip is situated in the bladder. If, however, doubt remains then remove the catheter and discuss with a urologist.

Tip Box
Antibiotic cover is likely to be required when changing a catheter due to catheter-associated urinary tract infection. Consult with local protocols or microbiology for advice as to specific antimicrobials.

POST-PROCEDURE INVESTIGATIONS

- Catheter sample urine for urine dip and microscopy, culture and sensitivity.
- Urine output on a fluid balance chart.

COMPLICATIONS

- Local discomfort – offer topical lidocaine gel and simple oral analgesia.
- Haematuria (secondary to local trauma).

- Catheter-associated urinary tract infection (or abscess formation reported with large-gauge catheters).
- Stricture formation or the formation of a false passage.
- Slowing of urine/no urine post catheter insertion:
  — secondary to catheter blockage (e.g. debris from pyuria or excess anaesthetic gel occluding catheter tip)
  — empty bladder
  — haematuria (clots blocking catheter).

In these circumstances consider flushing the catheter with 50 mL sterile normal saline or a three-way catheter (see Tip Boxes).

LUMBAR PUNCTURE

In 1885 the American neurologist James Leonard Corning (1855–1923) performed a lumbar puncture on a dog and injected cocaine in what proved to be the first demonstration of spinal anaesthesia. Heinrick Quincke (1842–1922) of Quincke's sign fame (capillary nailbed pulsation of aortic regurgitation) reported a lumbar puncture performed in 1888 for hydrocephalus-associated headaches 1 month before Walter Essex Wynter's (1860–1945) publication in the Lancet in 1889. Wynter described four cases of cerebrospinal fluid (CSF) aspiration in children with TB meningitis at the Middlesex Hospital, London which he performed by cut down to dura at L2 and placement of Southey's tubes for drainage.

INTRODUCTION

Lumbar puncture in the ward-based setting is usually performed in order to obtain CSF for investigation of neuroaxial conditions. Lumbar puncture is also commonly undertaken in order to provide spinal anaesthesia for operative procedures on the lower abdomen and lower limbs. Additionally lumbar puncture may be used for delivering intrathecal chemotherapy. However, these latter two situations are outside the remit of this chapter.

INDICATIONS

- Suspected central nervous system infection, e.g. meningitis.
- Suspected subarachnoid haemorrhage.
- Demyelination, e.g. multiple sclerosis.
- Meningeal carcinomatosis.
- Therapeutic reduction of CSF, e.g. benign intracranial hypertension.

CONTRAINDICATIONS

- Coagulopathy (recent aspirin, heparin last 12 hours, international normalized ratio above 1.2, activated partial thromboplastin time ratio above 1.2).
- Local sepsis over puncture site.
- Raised intracranial pressure (see Tip Box).
- Cardiorespiratory compromise.
- Suspected spinal cord mass or intracranial lesion (see Tip Box).
- Spinal cord compression.
- Lack of consent.
- Spinal cord deformities are a relative contraindication depending upon the spinal anatomy and the experience of the operator (e.g. scoliosis). If you are unsure of the anatomy, consult a senior colleague.

Tip Box

When to perform a head CT prior to lumbar puncture:

- >60 years of age.
- Symptoms or signs of raised intracranial pressure (persistent vomiting, history of recent seizure(s), reduced Glasgow coma scale, papilloedema).
- Focal abnormal neurology on examination.
- Immunocompromised (e.g. HIV positive).
- Recent head injury.
- When a possible intracranial bleed is the preliminary diagnosis (in which case a negative computerized tomography of the head should precede subsequent lumbar puncture).

EQUIPMENT

- Skin pen.
- Dressing pack.
- Sterile gown, gloves and drapes.
- Chlorhexidine cleaning solution.
- Lidocaine.
- 10 mL syringe.
- Orange needle.
- Green needle.
- Gauze.
- Manometer.
- Spinal needles (22 or 20 G).

- Collection bottles, labels and tin foil.
- Plaster.

Tip Box

Lumbar puncture needles are divided into two types: 'atraumatic' needles (e.g. Sprotte or Whitacre) and typical 'cutting' needles (Quincke) (Fig. 19.1).

The 'non-cutting' tip of atraumatic needles is designed to part the dural fibres rather than shear them, and so upon removal of the needle from the dura a smaller hole remains than with a cutting needle. This reduces the amount of CSF loss post-lumbar puncture, and several randomized double-blind studies have been published showing that post-lumbar puncture headaches are reduced ten-fold when using atraumatic needles.

Given their non-cutting tip design, atraumatic needles do not puncture the skin as freely as a typical Quincke needle. They require an introducer needle to puncture the skin, through which the atraumatic needle is passed. If you go on to use atraumatic needles, familiarize yourself with the apparatus prior to use.

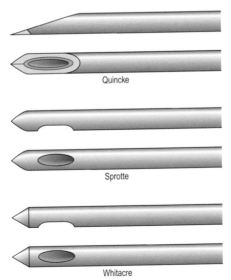

Quincke

Sprotte

Whitacre

Fig. 19.1   Atraumatic (e.g. Sprotte and Whitacre) and cutting (e.g. Quincke) needles used for lumbar puncture.

STRUCTURES THROUGH WHICH THE SPINAL NEEDLE PASSES

The lumbar puncture needle passes through the following tissues in sequence to reach the subarachnoid space (Fig. 19.2): skin, subcutaneous tissue, the supraspinal ligament, the interspinal ligament, the ligamentum flavum, the dura mater and finally the arachnoid mater.

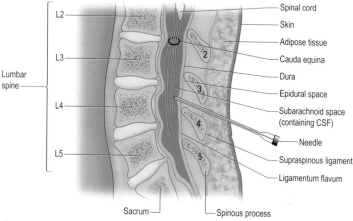

Fig. 19.2 Lumbar spinal anatomy.

PRACTICAL PROCEDURE

- Obtain consent.
- Provide analgesia, e.g. paracetamol or codeine.

POSITIONING

Correct positioning of the patient is paramount in successfully performing a lumbar puncture.

- Lateral decubitus/'foetal' position – Ensuring that the bed is flat, ask the patient to lie on their left side with their back flat to the edge of the bed and their shoulders square to their hips. Ensure that their knees are drawn into their chest and head tucked to chin to help open up the spinous processes. Once in position place a pillow under the head of the patient. It is also often helpful to have a pillow between the legs to avoid pelvic rotation, the aim being to ensure that the patient's back is flat flush to the edge of the bed.
- Seated position – This position is normally used in the event of a failed procedure in the lateral decubitus position. It has the advantage that there is less distortion of

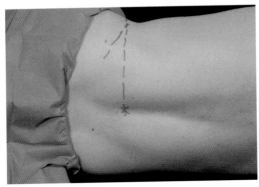

Fig. 19.3 Drop a vertical line down from most superior aspect of the iliac crest and mark the spine with a skin pen at the intersecting intervertebral space.

spinal anatomy, but with the disadvantage that the CSF pressure cannot be reliably ascertained in this position. Ask the patient to sit on the edge of the bed holding a pillow into their chest so that their spine is flexed forwards. Place their feet on a stool and point their chin to their chest to maximize spinal flexion. Alternatively, ask them to straddle a chair and lean onto a pillow ensuring the spine is flexed so the intervertebral spaces are open adequately.

The lower border of the spinal cord ends at the level of L1–2 at the conus medullaris. To ensure no damage to the cord, the spinal needle is inserted into the L3–4 intervertebral space. With the patient in the correct position, palpate the vertebral column at the L3–4 intervertebral space by joining an imaginary vertical line between the iliac crests across the back (Fig. 19.3). Mark this space with a skin pen so that it is clearly indicated.

Tip Box

Should you fail to obtain CSF via the L3–4 interspace, try one intervertebral space higher at L2–3.

PROCEDURE

- Number the specimen pots sequentially prior to specimen collection.
- Wash your hands, wear the sterile gown and gloves and lay out sterile environment and dressing pack.
- Check equipment:
  — Ensure the needle and metal stylet can be removed easily from one another and that the end of the needle fits the manometer.

— Familiarize yourself with the manometer directions ('open and closed to the patient' and 'neutral position'), and assemble the manometer with the 3-way tap turned to the 'closed to you' direction.

Tip Box

The 3-way tap is frequently very stiff for the initial few attempts at turning it and can consequently be cumbersome to manipulate during the procedure. For this reason, manipulate and loosen the 3-way tap between these positions several times prior to use.

- Clean the lumbar area – remember to clean spirally outwards from the central target to the periphery to avoid bringing dirty solution in contact with a previously cleaned area. Ensure that all cleaning fluid is wiped away prior to needle insertion.
- Place a drape over the iliac crest, enabling palpation of anatomical landmarks during the procedure whilst remaining sterile.
- Ensure you are comfortable. Most doctors sit on a chair, as standing in a very flexed position (especially if you are tall) is awkward and less controlled. Alter the bed height to help your personal comfort.
- Infiltrate local anaesthetic subcutaneously with an orange needle.
- Infiltrate local anaesthetic with a green needle between the spinous processes, to a maximum depth of approximately 2 cm.

Tip Box

Allow sufficient time for the anaesthetic block to take effect. If the superficial tissues are appropriately anaesthetized, lumbar puncture should be a painless procedure.

- Feel the disc interspace at level L3–4 and slowly insert the lumbar puncture needle bevel-up, pointing towards the patient's umbilicus.
- Check that the needle is in the midline and at 90 degrees to the skin while the pelvis remains perpendicular to the bed.

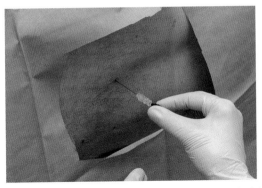

Fig. 19.4   Remove the stylet approximately every 3 mm you advance to check for CSF.

- Advance the needle for the first 2 cm, and thereafter periodically remove the stylet for approximately every 3 mm you advance (Fig. 19.4) to check for CSF (or blood if a venous plexus has been hit – in this case remove the needle).
- You may feel slight resistance passing through the ligamentum flavum before a 'push/give' through the dura into the subarachnoid space (usually at around 5–8 cm deep from the skin depending upon body habitus).
- On removing the stylet you will note CSF backflow through the needle. The CSF flow will depend on the gauge of the needle. The flow should be continuous. It might be initially blood stained but should clear (unless the diagnosis is subarachnoid haemorrhage).
- CSF opening pressure is measured by attaching the manometer (Fig. 19.5). This should be done as soon as one is satisfied that the CSF flow is continuous, although too much CSF free flow and loss will reduce the CSF pressure. Allow CSF to rise through the manometer until it completely stops rising. Record this level post-procedure.
- Switch the manometer to the 'closed to patient' direction and collect the first 5–10 drops of CSF in container 1.
- Remove the manometer and collect further samples of CSF in the corresponding numbered bottles, collecting 5–10 drops of CSF in each bottle (Fig. 19.6).
- When collected, replace the stylet and slowly remove the needle. Place a plaster over the site.
- Lie the patient on their back for an hour, remind them that they may feel light-headed or have a headache post-procedure.
- Prescribe analgesia, encourage oral fluid intake (if poor intake consider intravenous fluids, especially as the patient is lying flat).
- Document the procedure clearly in the patient's medical notes.

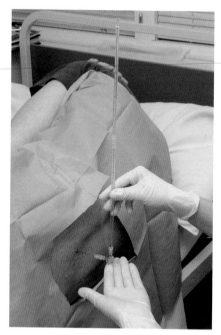

Fig. 19.5   Attaching the manometer once the CSF flow is continuous.

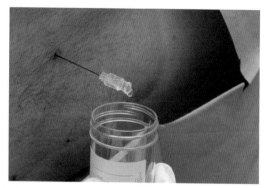

Fig. 19.6   Collect 5–10 drops of CSF in each bottle.

Tip Box

- If you are having trouble getting into the subarachnoid space (i.e. a dry tap), try rotating the needle, pulling the needle back or manoeuvring the needle slowly into different positions. If this fails, try the L2–3 interspace or move the patient into another position (see positioning above).
- If you hit bone or the patient experiences pain, slowly withdraw slightly and change the horizontal angle of trajectory of the needle.
- The amount of CSF needed by each laboratory varies. CSF cell count can be achieved with a few drops. However, virology, microbiology and cytology usually require at least 10 drops.
- It is prudent to take an extra specimen bottle for a spare CSF sample to save for any retrospective investigations or tests that require a large volume of CSF (and thus avoid a repeated lumbar puncture).

POST-PROCEDURE INVESTIGATIONS

Use a clear specimen bottle unless stated otherwise.

- Macroscopic appearance of CSF (normal is 'gin clear').
- CSF opening pressure (recorded on manometer).
- Cell count – white blood cell (including differential) and red blood cell counts.

Tip Box

In suspected subarachnoid haemorrhage, send bottles one and three for cell count. If the red blood cell count falls from bottle one to three this suggests a traumatic tap rather than blood truly within the CSF.

- Xanthochromia – spectrophotometry of sequential samples. The container should be shielded from external light by wrapping it in tin foil.
- CSF smear, Gram stain, MC+S, cell count – culture for bacteria, fungi, acid-fast bacilli (AFB).
- Glucose – in fluoride–oxalate tube. Send a concurrent serum glucose sample for accurate interpretation of the CSF glucose result (i.e. paired with CSF glucose).
- Protein and lactate dehydrogenase (LDH) levels.
- Viral PCR.
- Cytology.

SECTION 4   **Miscellaneous**

- Electrophoresis for oligoclonal bands.
- India ink stain for *Cryptococcus neoformans*.
- Treponemal titres for neurosyphilis.

COMPLICATIONS

- Post-procedure headache.
- Traumatic puncture.
- Puncture of lumbar veins.
- Subdural haematoma.
- Subarachnoid haemorrhage.
- Infection (meningitis).
- Epidural haematoma.

SUGGESTED READING

Kleyweg RP, Hertzberger LI, Carbaat PA et al (1998) Significant reduction in post-lumbar puncture headache using an atraumatic needle. A double-blind, controlled clinical trial. Cephalalgia 18(9): 635–7, discussion 591.

Müller B, Adelt K, Reichmann H, Toyka K (1994) Atraumatic needle reduces the incidence of post-lumbar puncture syndrome. J Neurol 241(6): 376–80.

Strupp M, Schueler O, Straube A et al (2001) "Atraumatic" Sprotte needle reduces the incidence of post-lumbar puncture headaches. Neurology 57(12): 2310–12.

ARTHROCENTESIS OF THE KNEE

The *Libellus de Medicinalibus Indorum Herbis* (or 'little book of the medicinal herbs of the Indians', originally an Aztec herbal manuscript composed in 1552 in Nahuatl which was translated into Latin) described puncturing the swollen joint with the bone of an eagle or a lion. The original book no longer exists but its translation was presented as a gift to Prince Philip (the future Philip II) of Spain. However, after several further owners and via a circuitous route over the centuries it ended up in the Vatican library. In 1990 Pope John Paul II returned it to Mexico.

INTRODUCTION

The aspiration and examination of fluid from the knee is fundamental to the investigation of an acute knee monoarthritis. The technique employed in arthrocentesis may also be employed for therapeutic purposes, although these should be performed by a specialist (rheumatologist or orthopaedic surgeon).

INDICATIONS

DIAGNOSTIC

The acutely swollen knee:

- Septic arthritis.
- Haemarthrosis.
- Gout.
- Pseudogout.

THERAPEUTIC

Only to be performed by a specialist:

- Intra-articular steroid or local anaesthetic administration (contraindicated in a suspected or confirmed septic joint).
- Drainage of a tense haemarthrosis.
- Drainage of a septic joint.

CONTRAINDICATIONS

- Lack of consent.
- Coagulopathy (should be corrected before aspiration to reduce the risk of haemarthrosis).
- Skin infection at the intended puncture site.
- Joint prosthesis (discuss the case with an orthopaedic surgeon).

EQUIPMENT

- Sterile gloves.
- Dressing pack.
- Chlorhexidine cleaning solution.
- Skin pen.
- Gauze.
- Orange needle.
- 2 × Green needle.
- 5 mL syringe.
- 20 mL syringe.
- Lidocaine.
- 3 × specimen pots.
- 1 × fluoride oxalate blood Vacutainer® (glucose).

PRACTICAL PROCEDURE

- Explain the procedure to the patient and obtain consent.
- Position the patient on a couch with the knee supported over pillows. This enables the quadriceps muscles to relax and the knee to be supported in a mildly flexed position, thus opening up the knee joint.
- Wash your hands and wear sterile gloves.
- Prepare the equipment on a sterile trolley.
- Clean the area – remember to clean outwards from the proposed site of aspiration (spirally from centre to periphery to avoid bringing dirty solution in contact with a previously cleaned area) to keep a clean field.

- The procedure is most commonly performed from the lateral approach. Palpate the knee joint, identifying the patella and in particular its most supero-lateral aspect. Mark the point 1 cm above and 1 cm lateral to the supero-lateral aspect of the patella (Fig. 20.1).
- Fill the 5 mL syringe with lidocaine via a green needle.
- Infiltrate local anaesthetic subcutaneously at the point identified above with an orange needle.
- Now infiltrate local anaesthetic with a green needle into deeper tissues, advancing the needle slowly at a 45 degree angle infero-medially under the patella until you aspirate fluid (Fig. 20.2). You may feel a slight 'give' as the needle enters the joint cavity. Allow a few minutes for the anaesthetic to take effect.

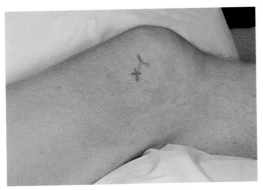

Fig. 20.1 Mark the point 1 cm above and 1 cm lateral to the supero-lateral aspect of the patella.

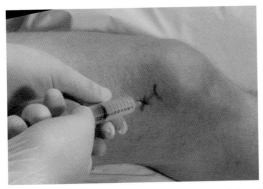

Fig. 20.2 Advance the needle slowly at a 45 degree angle infero-medially under the patella until you aspirate fluid.

Tip Box

If the patient experiences pain or there is resistance, the needle may be hitting the highly innervated periosteal or cartilaginous surfaces. Simply withdraw the needle slightly and realign the angle or direction of your subsequent approach.

Tip Box

If you cannot aspirate synovial fluid, try changing the position of the needle. Gently withdraw the needle and insert at a different angle aiming infero-medially behind the patella. Alternatively, change the position of the patient. Ask them to sit on the edge of a bed with their feet on a stool or on a chair. This opens up the articulating surfaces a little more to gain access to the joint.

- Attach a clean green needle to the 20 mL syringe. Insert the needle at the point 1 cm above and 1 cm lateral to the supero-lateral aspect of the patella and advance along the same anaesthetized track (directed at a 45 degree angle infero-medially under the patella) whilst aspirating to confirm entry to the synovium.
- Gently aspirate the synovial fluid either until the required volume for investigations is obtained, or to dryness for symptomatic relief.

Tip Box

Once the needle has entered the joint cavity, resistance to further aspiration or an apparently premature cessation of aspiration may result from turbid synovial fluid containing fibrin strands or debris. Try withdrawing the needle slightly and re-aspirate, or inject a small volume of synovial fluid to clear the needle. Alternatively, a larger-bore needle may be required to aspirate thick exudative effusions.

Tip Box

Compress the suprapatellar pouch, the patella itself and the medial aspect of the joint with your non-dominant hand whilst aspirating the knee to aid arthrocentesis and thus fully drain the joint effusion.

Tip Box

Having drained the synovial fluid, take care that when the joint surfaces come into apposition the needle tip does not cause local trauma.

- When enough synovial fluid has been obtained, withdraw the needle and place a small plaster over the puncture site.
- Prescribe adequate analgesia.

POST-PROCEDURE INVESTIGATIONS

- Macroscopic appearances:
  - Normal or non-inflammatory states – clear, straw-coloured fluid.
  - Haemarthrosis – bloody fluid.
  - Septic arthritis – cloudy, turbid fluid.
  - Inflammatory arthritis (crystal arthropathy, rheumatoid arthritis) – cloudy, turbid fluid.
- Microbiology:
  - Cell count – raised white cells (neutrophils) in septic arthritis and crystal arthropathies.
  - Gram stain.
  - Microscopy, culture and sensitivity.
  - Alcohol- and acid-fast bacilli + Ziehl–Nielson/Auramine staining.
- Biochemistry:
  - Protein – high (>4 g/dL) in inflammatory or purulent effusions.
  - Glucose (with concurrent serum glucose sample) – comparatively low to serum glucose in inflammatory or purulent effusions.
  - LDH – high in inflammatory or purulent effusions.
- Microscopy under polarized light (for crystal arthropathies):
  - Gout – negatively bi-refringent needle-like crystals.
  - Pseudogout – weekly positive bi-refringent rhomboidal crystals.

COMPLICATIONS

- Bleeding (either superficial or intra-articular).
- Infection (either superficial or intra-articular) – a rare complication when strict aseptic technique is observed, although much increased when overlying infection (a contraindication to arthrocentesis) is present.
- Dry tap.
- Pain.

SUBCUTANEOUS AND INTRAMUSCULAR INJECTIONS

The Irish physician Francis Rynd (1811–1861) invented the hollow needle in 1844, patented in the Irish patents office. Charles Gabriel Pravaz (1791–1853), a French physician, created the first hypodermic tubular needle and syringe in 1853, made entirely from silver. Soon after, the Scottish physician Alexander Wood (1817–1884) went on to develop a method for subcutaneous injection. Not without an unfortunate sense of irony, the first recorded fatality from an overdose administered by Wood's invention was that of his wife who had become addicted to intravenous morphine.

INTRODUCTION

Subcutaneous and intramuscular injections provide routes for medication delivery that do not require intravenous access. This may be advantageous in either an emergency situation (e.g. intramuscular epinephrine) or electively (e.g. subcutaneous insulin).

INDICATIONS

- Subcutaneous injections, e.g. insulin, tetracosactide, growth hormone, morphine sulphate.
- Intramuscular injections, e.g. haloperidol, epinephrine, metoclopramide, cyclizine.

CONTRAINDICATIONS

- Local contraindications to injection include:
  — cellulitis
  — haematoma
  — lipoatrophy
  — lipohypertrophy
  — lymphoedema.
- Bleeding diatheses – coagulopathy or thrombocytopaenia may increase the risk of subcutaneous or intramuscular haematoma formation.
- Lack of consent.

Tip Box

Under common law intramuscular sedation in the acutely confused patient does not require the patient's consent if:

- the patient lacks capacity and
- the administration of the medication is in the best interests of the patient (and not those of the ward staff!)

This route for delivery of sedative medications does not work instantly, and the need for it should be carefully considered prior to prescription.

EQUIPMENT

- Gloves.
- Sterile hypodermic needles (Fig. 21.1):
  — 25 gauge needle (orange: length 16 mm, inner diameter 0.241 mm) for subcutaneous delivery
  — 21 gauge (green: length 40 mm, inner diameter 0.495 mm) to 23 gauge needle (blue: length 30 mm, inner diameter 0.318 mm) for intramuscular delivery
  — 21 gauge needle for drawing up the drug.
- Syringe (of required volume for the medication +/– volume of dilutant required to reconstitute the medication).
- Sterile alcohol swabs.
- Gauze.
- Plaster.
- Vial of medication to be administered. Always read the instructions to check the correct dosage, route of delivery and solution required to reconstitute the powder form of the medication.
- Sharps bin.

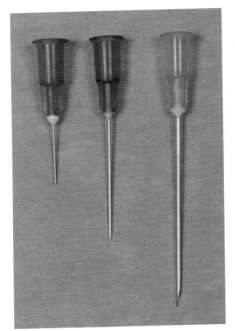

Fig. 21.1 Hypodermic needles have standard colour coding according to their gauge.

PRACTICAL PROCEDURE

PREPARATION

- Explain the procedure to the patient and gain consent.
- Position the patient and expose the area for injection.
- Wash your hands and wear gloves.
- Perform the following checks prior to administering any medication:
  — Confirm the patient's personal details and check that they correspond with their drug chart and name band.
  — On the drug chart confirm the patient's drug allergies, the drug to be given, the dose required, the timing of the dose and the route of administration.
  — Check the drug itself together with the dosage and expiry date in the presence of a colleague.
- Draw up the required volume of specified dilutant (see information accompanying the medication) into the syringe using a green needle.
- Open the vial of medication for injection. Insert the syringe containing the dilutant attached to the green needle. Insert a second green needle into the vial to allow air to escape when adding dilutant.

- Reconstitute the medication in the vial and aspirate into the syringe when complete. Discard the vial and green needles into a sharps bin.
- Expel any excess air or air bubbles from the syringe by gently tapping the side of the syringe whilst holding it upright.
- Clean the area of skin for injection with sterile alcohol swabs and allow to dry.

Tip Box

Allowing the alcohol to evaporate from the skin surface is the mechanism of its bacteriocidal activity, not the vigour with which you clean the area! Furthermore, injecting before the alcohol has evaporated is more painful for the patient.

SUBCUTANEOUS INJECTION

- Attach the 25 gauge (orange) needle to the syringe.
- Choose a site for injection. Suitable sites include the triceps area, anterior thigh area or the abdomen.
- Pinch and lift the skin overlying this area gently into a fold between the thumb and index finger of your non-dominant hand, thereby separating the subcutaneous adipose tissue layer from the muscle (Fig. 21.2).
- Warn the patient of a sharp scratch.
- Gently insert needle into the skin at a 30–45 degree angle.

Tip Box

When injecting with a shorter needle, such as when administering insulin, a 90 degree angle is the most appropriate approach for insertion.

- Slowly inject the medication.

Tip Box

For subcutaneous medication delivery you do not need to aspirate prior to injection. Aspiration may in fact predispose to haematoma formation when administering subcutaneous heparin.

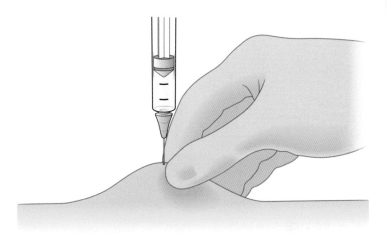

Fig. 21.2   Pinch and lift the skin into a fold, separating the subcutaneous adipose tissue layer from the muscle.

INTRAMUSCULAR INJECTION

- Attach the 23 gauge (blue) or 21 gauge (green) needle to the syringe.

Tip Box

Needle size will be influenced by the patient's body habitus. In obese individuals intramuscular injection in the buttock will require the length of a green needle.

- Choose a site for injection taking into account the individual's muscle mass. Suitable muscles include the deltoids, the gluteal muscles and the lateral thigh muscles.

Tip Box

When injecting into the gluteal muscles, split the buttock into four quadrants (Fig. 21.3). Only inject into the upper outer quadrant to minimize the risk of sciatic nerve injury.

- Pull the skin taught over the underlying muscle layer and insert the needle in one swift motion.

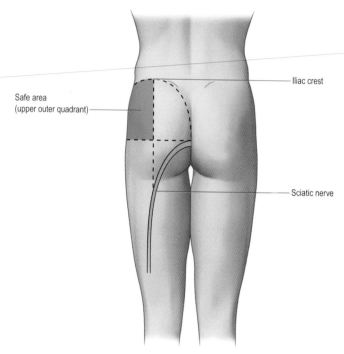

Iliac crest

Safe area
(upper outer quadrant)

Sciatic nerve

Fig. 21.3 Use the upper outer quadrant of the buttock to avoid sciatic nerve injury.

Tip Box

This technique is termed the 'Z track'. Upon releasing the tension applied to the overlying skin, the needle track from the skin to the underlying muscle disappears and hence reduces the risk of medication leakage through the puncture site following the injection.

- Aspirate the syringe to ensure that the needle is not in a blood vessel.
- Slowly inject the medication at a rate of approximately 1 mL every 10 seconds. This allows the muscle fibres to expand, thus preventing pain and ensuring an even distribution of the drug.

FINISHING OFF

- Remove the needle and apply pressure to the puncture site with gauze or cotton wool to prevent haematoma formation.
- Dispose of the syringe and needle into a sharps bin.
- Attach a plaster if needed.
- Observe for any adverse drug reactions.
- Record the date and time of injection on the patient's drug chart.

Tip Box

Rotate injection sites to minimize the risks of infection (either superficial cellulitis or deep abscess formation), atrophy and hypertrophy of the underlying tissue.

COMPLICATIONS

- Local infection – either superficial (cellulitis) or deep (abscess formation).
- Bleeding – either superficial or deep haematoma formation. This may predispose to infection.
- Lipoatrophy.
- Lipohypertrophy.
- Injection fibrosis – if injections are delivered with an incorrect technique or too frequently to that site.

LOCAL ANAESTHETICS

Sigmund Freud was aware of the analgesic properties of cocaine, but its anaesthetic properties were recognized by his colleague, the Austrian ophthalmologist Karl Koller (1857–1944). He successfully performed eye surgery utilizing the local anaesthetic properties of cocaine in 1884, a significant breakthrough in the developing field of anaesthesia.

INTRODUCTION

Local anaesthetic agents have varying onset times, duration of action and ability to penetrate tissue. Chemically they are separated into esters (cocaine, procaine, amethocaine) and amides (lidocaine, prilocaine, bupivacaine), which is relevant to their metabolism and tendency to toxicity. Esters are rapidly metabolized by serum and liver cholinesterase and therefore metabolism is retarded by low enzyme levels such as pregnancy or liver disease. Amides are metabolized by liver microsomal enzymes, which may be less effective when hepatic function or blood flow are reduced.

Local anaesthetics work by reversibly blocking conduction along nerve fibres through binding to voltage-gated sodium channels in the neuronal membrane. This prevents sodium ion entry during depolarization, which in turn prevents the propagation of the action potential. The membrane in effect becomes stabilized. Consequently, the response to painful stimuli is not effected and pain is not sensed centrally.

Local anaesthetics are weak bases and are most efficacious in alkaline conditions, whereby the un-ionized form crosses the neuronal membrane. Conversely, infected or inflamed tissues have an acidic environment, which reduces the action of local anaesthetics. Furthermore, the increased vascularity of these environments gives rise to an increased risk of systemic absorption and subsequent side-effects. Local anaesthetics affect the smaller nerves such as the autonomic before the medium-sized sensory and large motor nerves. They are more effective at higher concentrations, having a shorter onset and longer duration. The duration of local anaesthetics is prolonged when combined with vasoconstrictors such as weak epinephrine solutions (e.g. 1 in 200,000).

INDICATIONS

These anaesthetics provide local anaesthesia for painful procedures. The most commonly used local anaesthetic for ward-based procedures is lidocaine (also known as lignocaine). Various lidocaine preparations are available:

- Topical cream – anaesthesia before minor skin procedures, e.g. cannulation.
- Topical gel – e.g. catheterization.
- Injection – e.g. central line insertion, chest and ascitic drain insertion, lumbar puncture, suturing.
- Injection in combination with epinephrine prolongs the local anaesthetic effect by reducing blood flow and thus the rate of systemic absorption. However, this is usually required in specialist circumstances such as facial or scalp anaesthesia, and is not recommended for use in the procedures described in this book.

DOSAGE

The concentration of lidocaine (mg/mL) equals the percentage concentration multiplied by 10. For example:

- 1% lidocaine = 10 mg/mL.
- 2% lidocaine = 20 mg/mL.

The maximum dose of lidocaine (without vasoconstrictor agent) can be calculated as follows:

$$\text{Maximum dose (mg) of lidocaine} = 3 \times \text{weight (kg)}$$

- For example, for an individual weighing:

70 kg, maximum dose lidocaine = 210 mg (21 mL 1%, or 10.5 mL 2%).

55 kg, maximum dose lidocaine = 165 mg (16.5 mL 1%, or 8.25 mL 2%).

Tip Box
The British National Formulary (BNF) recommends to reduce the dose in elderly or debilitated patients when using local anaesthetics.

COMPLICATIONS – LIDOCAINE TOXICITY

The membrane-stabilizing effects of local anaesthetics can become excessive if plasma concentrations become elevated. This leads to toxic effects, particularly affecting neural and cardiovascular tissues. The permitted dosage should therefore be strictly adhered to.

- Arterial plasma concentrations of local anaesthetic (through local absorption and uptake into the systemic circulation) peak within about 10–30 minutes. Toxic effects are most likely to manifest during this period.
- Initial side-effects include a feeling of 'light-headedness', circumoral paraesthesia, visual disturbances and twitching.
- More severe toxic effects include convulsions, cardiac arrhythmias and cardiovascular collapse. These can occur rapidly upon inadvertent intravascular administration.
- The management of these toxic effects would be in accordance with the Resuscitation Council (UK) guidelines for adult advanced life support (ALS).
- Intravenous benzodiazepines not only have a role in seizure termination but also in raising seizure threshold. They should therefore be considered in the prevention of seizures when frequent twitching is observed.

Tip Box

The British National Formulary (BNF) recommends that when using local anaesthetics 'resuscitative equipment should be available'.

CONTRAINDICATIONS

- Complete heart block.
- Certain arrhythmogenic cardiological conditions are exacerbated by local anaesthetics (e.g. bupivacaine in Brugada syndrome). Consult with a specialist before using local anaesthetics in these patients.
- Hypovolaemia.
- Known allergy to lidocaine (rare).
- Local anaesthetic in combination with epinephrine should NEVER be used in digits and appendages given the consequent risk of ischaemic necrosis.

PRACTICAL PROCEDURE

FIELD BLOCK

This is used for anaesthesia of small cutaneous nerves.

- Explain the procedure to the patient and gain consent.
- Wash your hands and wear sterile gloves.
- Prepare the site of the procedure using sterile technique.

Tip Box

Initial subcutaneous infiltration of local anaesthetic gives rise to a small wheal or bleb, which commonly distorts the anatomical landmarks at the site of the intended procedure. It is therefore useful to mark such landmarks with a skin pen prior to infiltration.

- Ask an assistant to show you the vial of local anaesthetic prior to drawing it up. Check the date, concentration and drug name on the vial.
- To maintain aseptic technique, the assistant opens the vial of local anaesthetic and offers it to the operator's needle.
- Attach a small-calibre needle (such as an orange needle) to the syringe for initial skin and subcutaneous infiltration.
- Warn the patient of a sharp scratch and a subsequent stinging sensation prior to administration.
- Take care to avoid accidental intravascular injection: ALWAYS draw back on the syringe prior to infiltrating.
- Infiltrate deeper tissues with a green needle.

Tip Box

Allow a few minutes for subcutaneous anaesthesia to take effect, then ensure adequate anaesthesia by testing for sensation with either ethyl chloride spray or a needle tip prior to performing the intended procedure.

DIGITAL BLOCK

Each digit is innervated by two dorsal and two ventral nerve branches (Fig. 22.1). Anaesthesia of a digit (e.g. prior to cleaning a digital wound or manipulating a digital fracture) can be performed either by a ring block or a tendon (transthecal) block.

Tip Box

When performing a digital block, ALWAYS check for neurovascular integrity (i.e. examine perfusion and sensation) prior to administering local anaesthetic.

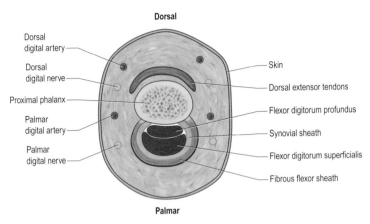

Fig. 22.1   Digital anatomy in cross-section.

RING BLOCK

- Position the patient's hand with fingers extended and abducted.
- Insert the needle into the dorsolateral aspect of the digit at the level of the base of the metacarpal bone and administer approximately 1 mL of 1% lidocaine local anaesthetic (Fig. 22.2).
- Repeat this procedure at the same point on the opposite side of the digit.
- Wait a few minutes to allow the local anaesthetic to diffuse through the subcutaneous tissue and infiltrate the dorsal and ventral nerve branches.

TENDON (TRANSTHECAL) BLOCK

In tendon block local anaesthetic is infused along the flexor tendon sheath.

- Inject between 2–3 mL of 1% lidocaine into the flexor tendon at the base of the digit (Fig. 22.3).

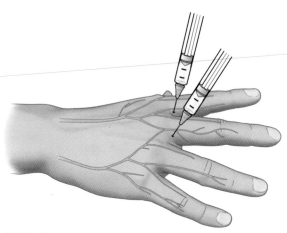

Fig. 22.2 With the fingers extended and abducted, insert the needle into the dorsolateral aspect of the digit at the level of the base of the metacarpal bone.

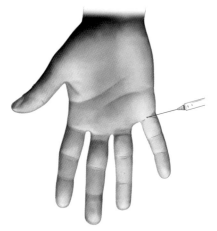

Fig. 22.3 Inject local anaesthetic into the flexor tendon sheath at the base of the digit.

SUTURING

Prior to his post as physician to the Emperor Marcus Aurelius, the Greek physician Galen (129–circa 200–216) worked for several years gaining experience in the management of trauma as physician in a gladiator school. There he described using sutures for the purposes of haemostasis and tendon repair.

Lord Joseph Lister (1827–1912) introduced sutures treated with carbolic acid to promote antisepsis, as well as pioneering the process of chromatization to prolong the tensile strength of the suture. In these times suture material was most commonly derived from violin strings, the instrument itself being referred to as the 'kit' (from the word 'kitara', what we now refer to as the guitar). The intestines of the sheep, goat or ox were used to make these strings, termed 'kitgut'. Suture material subsequently became referred to as 'catgut' despite not using the intestines of the cat in their production.

INTRODUCTION

Suturing is a skill commonly required outside the operating theatre, especially in A&E for minor trauma. Prior to suturing, a careful neurovascular and motor examination is *always* required as well as examining the wound for debris or foreign bodies.

INDICATIONS

- Wound closure (healing by primary intention).
- Securing drains (e.g. chest or ascitic drains) or lines (e.g. central venous or arterial lines) to skin.

Tip Box

Always consider the alternatives to sutures when contemplating wound closure, including surgical staples, wound-closure adhesive tape (e.g. Steri-Strips®) and dermal adhesives (cyanoacrylate skin glues, e.g. Dermabond®).

CAUTIONS

Superficial skin lacerations are commonly managed in the A&E setting. However, always seek senior or expert guidance prior to suturing if unsure.

- Injuries to extremities that occurred over 12 hours prior to presentation may, following appropriate cleaning, be left to heal by secondary intention.
- Seek a specialist referral if, on examination, there is any evidence of underlying bone fracture or neurovascular or motor deficit relating to the injury.
- Plastic surgery specialists will consider referrals or will readily give advice for any cases involving skin wounds if required.
- In general, proceed with caution in cases in which the cosmetic outcome is of greater significance to the patient:
  — paediatric cases
  — maxillofacial cases.
- Caution should also be used with bites, either human or animal. Closed-fist bites (e.g. sustained when the patient's fist comes into contact with another person's teeth) can lead to deep tendon infections, and are worth discussing with orthopaedic or hand specialists. Animal bites, if superficial, may also require a senior opinion with respect to antibiotic prophylaxis.

CONTRAINDICATIONS

- Lack of consent.
- Foreign body in the wound.
- Wound infection.

Tip Box

Obtain an X-ray to look for glass, marking the soft tissue injury with a paper clip to highlight its position an the radiograph.

EQUIPMENT

- Sterile gloves and drapes.
- Chlorhexidine cleaning solution.
- 1 L bag of normal saline, giving set, sterile scissors and eye goggles.
- Lidocaine.
- 1 × 10 mL syringe.
- Orange needle.
- Green needle.
- Suture cutter.
- Suture pack (including toothed forceps, non-toothed forceps and needle holder).
- Gauze.
- Sterile dressing.
- Non-absorbable suture (e.g. '1' silk).
  - — Non-absorbable sutures may be made from silk, nylon, polypropylene (Prolene) or polyester (Dacron).
  - — Sutures are sized by the United States Pharmacopoeia (USP) scale (Table 23.1). For example, an 11-0 suture would be appropriate for specialist ophthalmic surgery, a 4-0/5-0 suture for closing a limb wound, and a 2-0 suture for securing a central venous catheter.
  - — Several types of needle points are in common use (e.g. cutting, atraumatic and taper-cutting needles). However, whether the needle shape is straight or curved is particularly important in simple suturing. Curved needles are designed for use with needle-holders, whereas straight needles are designed to be hand-held (thus concomitantly increasing the associated risk of needlestick injury).

PRACTICAL PROCEDURE

THE SIMPLE INTERRUPTED SUTURE

- Obtain consent.
- Ask a nurse to accompany you in order to open non-sterile equipment and to comfort the patient.
- Wash your hands, wear the sterile gloves and lay out sterile environment and suture pack.
- Inspect and clean the area. Closely inspect the inside of the wound for debris or foreign bodies. Irrigate the wound with copious volumes of sterile normal saline until you are satisfied that the wound is clean.

TABLE 23.1 United States Pharmacopoeia (USP) scale of suture sizes

Gauge (USP scale)	Non-absorbable suture diameter (mm)
11-0	0.01
10-0	0.02
9-0	0.03
8-0	0.04
7-0	0.05
6-0	0.07
5-0	0.10
4-0	0.15
3-0	0.20
2-0	0.30
0	0.35
1	0.40
2	0.50
3	0.60
4	0.60
5	0.70
6	0.80

Tip Box

'The solution to pollution is dilution'. Attach a giving set to a sterile 1 L bag of normal saline and cut off the lower two-thirds to half of the set using sterile scissors. Irrigate the wound liberally, squeezing the bag to direct a high-velocity jet of fluid directly into the wound. Always wear eye goggles when performing this technique and place a disposable absorbable pad and kidney bowl underneath the area being cleaned.

- Clean the surrounding skin outwards from the wound with chlorhexidine solution. Apply the sterile drape with only the wound exposed, giving a sterile field for suturing.
- Infiltrate local anaesthetic subcutaneously with an orange needle.
- Infiltrate local anaesthetic with a green needle into deeper tissues.
- Check that the area is satisfactorily anaesthetized.

- Grasp the needle with the needle-holder approximately three-quarters to two-thirds of its length from the needle point (Fig. 23.1).
- Starting at the middle of the wound, lift the distal skin edge with toothed forceps in the non-dominant hand and hold the needle-holder with the dominant hand in a pronated position (Fig. 23.2).
- Insert the needle at right angles to the skin approximately half to one centimetre from the wound edge and rotate the needle through the epidermis and dermis by supinating the dominant hand, thus rotating through the curvature of the needle. Ensure the needle passes through the bottom of the wound leaving no dead space

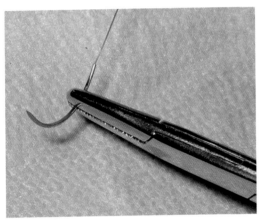

Fig. 23.1 Grasp the suture needle half to two-thirds along from the tip.

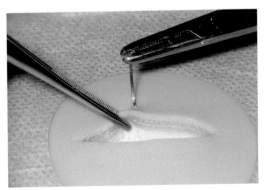

Fig. 23.2 Starting at the middle of the wound, lift the distal skin edge with toothed forceps and insert the needle at right angles to the skin approximately half to one centimetre from the wound edge.

deep to the suture. This secures a good 'bite' of healthy, undamaged skin and subcutaneous tissue (Fig. 23.3).

- Now release the needle from the needle-holder and re-grasp the needle within the wound cavity whilst continuing to keep the wound edge held open with the toothed forceps.
- Lift the proximal edge of the skin with the toothed forceps in the non-dominant hand. Again, hold the needle-holder with the dominant hand in a pronated position.
- Return the needle to the bottom of the wound and insert it perpendicularly into the subcutaneous tissue (Fig. 23.4).

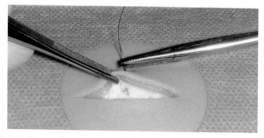

Fig. 23.3   Ensure the needle passes through the base of the wound.

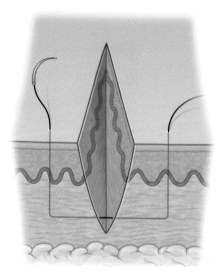

Fig. 23.4   Return the needle to the bottom of the wound and insert it perpendicularly into the subcutaneous tissue leaving no dead space deep to the suture.

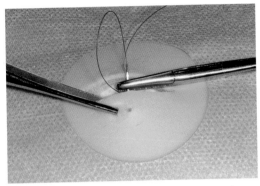

Fig. 23.5   Bring the needle out directly opposite and equidistant from the wound.

- Supinate the dominant wrist in order to keep the body of the needle perpendicular to the tissue it is passing through upwards to the skin surface. Aim to bring the needle through the skin at a point directly opposite and equidistant from the wound compared with the other side (Fig. 23.5).
- Pull the suture carefully through the wound by the needle. Leave approximately 5 cm of suture material free on the opposite side.

Tip Box

Pull the suture in line with the needle to avoid breaking the suture from the needle.

- Let go of the needle and close the needle holder whilst positioning it along the line of the wound.
- Coil the suture material around the needle holder twice in a clockwise motion (Fig. 23.6A and B).
- Open and turn the needle holder towards the free end of the suture. Grasp the free end.
- Pull the free end through the coils, keeping the suture as flat as possible to the skin. Pull the suture through so that the knot lays flat to the skin surface with the wound edges apposed to one another. Do not lie the knot over the wound, but to the side of it over the adjacent skin.

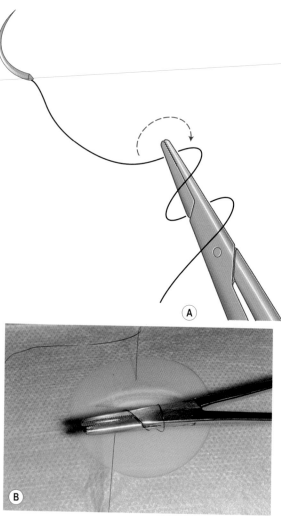

Fig. 23.6 (A) Coil the suture material around the needle holder twice in a clockwise motion. (B) Open the needle-holder to grasp the free end of the suture.

Tip Box
'Lock' the knot by pulling the knot in the direction of the wound (i.e. perpendicular to the suture).

Tip Box
Do not place the stitches so tight that the wound is under tension. The purpose of the stitch is to appose the wound edges.

- Now let go of the suture and again close the needle holder positioning it along the line of the wound.
- Repeat the coiling procedure twice more using only one coil each time and in alternate directions (i.e. anticlockwise for the first single throw, then clockwise for the second single throw, Fig. 23.7).
- Cut the suture at approximately 1 cm in length from the skin (to aid suture removal).
- Place further sutures at half to one centimetre intervals working outwards from the centre of the wound.
- Clean the area and apply a dry dressing.
- Document the procedure clearly in the patient's medical notes.

For further suture techniques see Fig. 23.8.

POST-PROCEDURE CARE

- Prescribe oral analgesia.
- Check patient's tetanus status and give booster if required.
- If required (e.g. animal bites) consider prophylactic antibiotics. Discuss this with microbiology/consult local protocols.
- Advise the patient to attend their GP for removal of sutures (ROS) at the suggested date (Table 23.2).
- Reassure the patient that stitch removal is a painless procedure.

Tip Box

Having inspected a wound prior to suture removal, only go on to remove the sutures from the healed area(s). Wound dehiscence may result from premature suture removal.

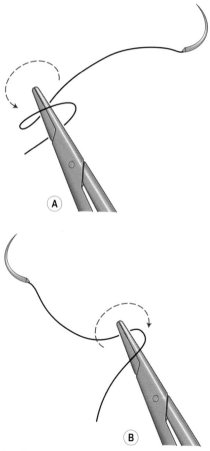

Fig. 23.7 (A) Coil the suture anticlockwise for the first single throw, then (B) clockwise for the second single throw.

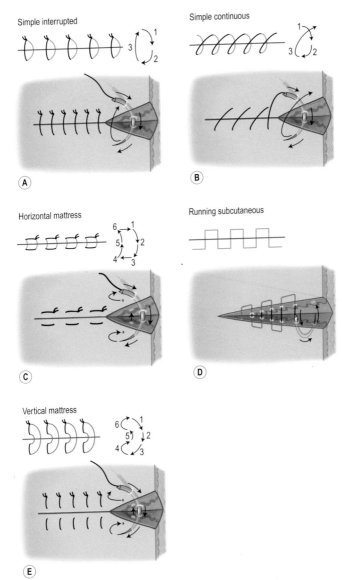

Fig. 23.8 (A) Simple interrupted sutures (as described). (B) Simple continuous.
(C) Horizontal mattress. (D) Running subcutaneous sutures. (E) Vertical mattress.

TABLE 23.2 Suggested dates for removal of sutures (ROS)

Suture location	ROS at day
Face and neck	3–5
Neck	5–8
Scalp	7–10
Trunk	10–14
Limbs	10–14
Foot	14–21

- Supply the patient with a wound care advice card. In general the patient should be advised to:
  - keep the wound clean and dry for at least 48 hours
  - seek medical attention if there is any evidence of infection, e.g. erythema, tenderness, discharge or swelling from the wound
  - avoid putting the wound under tension (for example, lifting heavy objects or contact sports) for up to 6 weeks.

COMPLICATIONS

- Infection.
- Failure of wound healing.
- Hypertrophic or keloid scarring (more common in younger individuals and those with pigmented skin).

INDEX

Note:
Page numbers in **bold** refer to major sections/discussions in the text

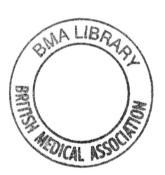